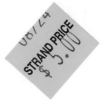

# Nutrition and
# Gastroenterology

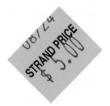

# CURRENT CONCEPTS IN NUTRITION

---

**Myron Winick, Editor**

*Institute of Human Nutrition*
*Columbia University College of Physicians and Surgeons*

# NUTRITION AND GASTROENTEROLOGY

*Edited by*

**MYRON WINICK**

*Institute of Human Nutrition*
*Columbia University College of Physicians and Surgeons*

A WILEY-INTERSCIENCE PUBLICATION

**JOHN WILEY & SONS**

New York • Chichester • Brisbane • Toronto

*Library of Congress Cataloging in Publication Data:*

Main entry under title:

Nutrition and gastroenterology.
   (Current concepts in nutrition ; v. 9 ISSN 0090-0443)
   Based on the Symposium on Nutrition and Gastroenterology held Nov. 1979 in New York.
   "A Wiley-Interscience publication."
   Includes index.
   1. Nutritionally induced diseases—Congresses.
2. Digestive organs—Diseases—Nutritional aspects—
Congresses.  3. Nutrition—Congresses.  4. Gastroenterology—Congresses.  I. Winick, Myron.  II. Symposium
on Nutrition and Gastroenterology, New York, 1979.
III. Series. [DNLM:  1. Gastroenterology—Congresses.
2. Nutrition—Congresses.  W1 CU788AS v. 9 / WI100

S9924n  1979]
RC622.N88      616.3      80-16169
ISBN 0-471-08173-6

Printed in the United States of America

10 9 8 7 6 5 4 3 2 1

*To the memory of **Dr. Daniel Kimberg**, Chairman of the Department of Medicine, College of Physicians & Surgeons of Columbia University.*

*Dr. Kimberg was a major planner of the Symposium on Nutrition and Gastroenterology, upon which this volume is based. He was a leading investigator in the field of gastroenterology and a dedicated physician and teacher. His untimely death a few days prior to the Symposium is a great loss to all who knew him. He will be missed by the entire medical community. We hope that the publication of this volume, the proceedings of the last scientific meeting in which he was involved, will contribute in some small way to perpetuating the memory of this great physician.*

# Preface

---

The purpose of this volume is to acquaint physicians and nutritionists with the latest research documenting the importance of the gastrointestinal tract in the maintenance of good nutrition and conversely the importance of good nutrition in maintaining proper gastrointestinal function.

The book is divided into three parts. The first discusses the process by which various nutrients are digested and absorbed. The second discusses the various diseases within the GI tract that can affect the digestion and absorption of nutrients, and the third considers the effects of various nutritional alterations on specific functions of the GI tract. Thus, not only is the importance of a properly functioning GI tract to adequate nutrition documented but also the importance of proper nutrition in maintaining adequate GI function is considered.

The authors of each chapter are experts in the areas they are covering and each has contributed significantly to our present understanding of the subject under discussion.

In Part 1, the structure of the GI tract, including its ultrastructure as it relates to the absorption of nutrients, is considered. This is followed by a detailed description of how fat, carbohydrate, protein, and minerals, particularly calcium, are absorbed through the GI tract. The mechanisms involved in the digestion and absorption of each of these nutrients are carefully outlined. The newest information is presented and the gaps in our present knowledge are pointed out.

In Part 2 malabsorption of various nutrients is considered in detail. In addition, such diseases as regional ileitis, ulcerative colitis, peptic ulcer, alcoholism and other diseases of the liver, and various surgical procedures are considered. The authors of these chapters discuss not only the abnormalities in absorption produced by these diseases but also the best available means of treatment.

Part 3 discusses how early nutrition affects the development of the GI tract and the ways by which malnutrition alters GI function. In the first case the importance of even the initial feedings in the proper development of GI structure and function is demonstrated. In the second, the devastating effects of severe malnutrition on specific GI functions are carefully detailed.

The book, I hope, will serve as a reference for those interested in one or more of these areas. In addition, however, and perhaps more important, it should supply a framework on which to build for those who must care for patients with nutritional or gastrointestinal disorders.

MYRON WINICK

*New York, New York*
*July 1980*

# Contents

**PART 3    EFFECT OF ALTERED NUTRITION
          ON THE GASTROINTESTINAL TRACT**

# PART 1

# Nutrient Absorption

# 1

# Structure of the Gastrointestinal Tract as it Relates to Nutrient Movement

SEYMOUR M. SABESIN, M.D.

University of Tennessee Center for the Health Sciences, and Veterans Administration Hospital, Memphis, Tennessee

Correlative biochemical and ultrastructural studies (1, 2) of the small intestinal epithelium have provided exciting new insights into the mechanisms by which these specialized cells regulate the absorption of specific nutrients while at the same time discriminating against the absorption of potentially noxious substances (e.g., foreign proteins). Furthermore, elegant ultrastructural studies (3, 4) utilizing newer morphological techniques, such as freeze fracture, enzyme histochemistry, and immunochemical techniques, combined with biochemical analysis of intestinal epithelial subcellular fractions, have defined the chemical composition of membrane components and thus have provided a biochemical and structural basis for the specificity of specific nutrient transport. Thus such studies have localized the disaccharidases and peptidases to the so-called "glycocalyx" of the microvilli (5), have shown that Na+, K+, ATPase is localized in the lateral-basal epithelial cell (6) membranes, and have suggested that carrier proteins for sugar and amino acid transport are also located in microvillus membranes facing the luminal surface (7). Information concerning the function of the smooth and rough endoplasmic reticulum and the Golgi apparatus in the biosynthesis and intracellular

Some of the research reported here was supported in part by NIH grant HL–23945 (formerly AM–17398) and by grants from the Veterans Administration, the American Heart Association, and the American Egg Board.

3

transport of chylomicrons during fat absorption has also been derived from morphological and biochemical investigations (8, 9).

Ultrastructural studies (10) have defined the morphology of the various junctional complexes between adjacent epithelial cells. Although membrane junctions are, of course, not confined to the intestinal epithelium, they have been extensively studied in this tissue and provide yet another example of the exquisite organization of the absorbing surface, since the junctional complexes knit individual epithelial cells into a syncytium which permits direct cell to cell communication through so-called "gap" junctions while preventing the loss of absorbed nutrients that have entered the intercellular space by forming areas of dense adhesion called tight junctions.

This chapter will describe the functional morphology of the intestinal epithelial absorptive cells, thereby providing the morphological basis for those chapters which will deal with the mechanisms of absorption of specific nutrients. In addition, the absorption of dietary triglycerides will be used to illustrate the role of subcellular organelles in the intracellular synthesis, transport, and secretion of one class of nutrients.

## NORMAL STRUCTURE OF THE SMALL INTESTINAL EPITHELIAL ABSORPTIVE CELLS

Nutrient absorption and transport by the small intestinal epithelium involves the movement of nutrients from the intestinal lumen across the barrier provided by the microvillus membrane into the cell and thence into the blood or lymph. To facilitate the rapidity and efficiency of absorption, the mucosa of the small intestine presents an enormous surface area which is enhanced by the formation of villi lined with epithelial cells. The villi measure 0.5–1.0 mm in height and increase the absorptive surface eightfold (11). The luminal surface of the columnar epithelial cells, which comprise the villi, contains specialized fingerlike projections called microvilli which are some $0.1~\mu$ wide and $0.7$–$1.5~\mu$ in height (11). The microvilli increase the absorptive surface enormously (14–39 times), and also provide a structural component through which all nutrients must pass before entering the intracellular compartment (Figure 1).

Adjacent absorptive cells are separated from each other by intricate interdigitations of their lateral plasma membranes (Figure 1). The cytoplasmic components are similar to those of other epithelial and glandular cells, containing components of smooth and rough endoplasmic reticulum, a well-defined Golgi complex, mitochondria, and lysosomes (Figure 1).

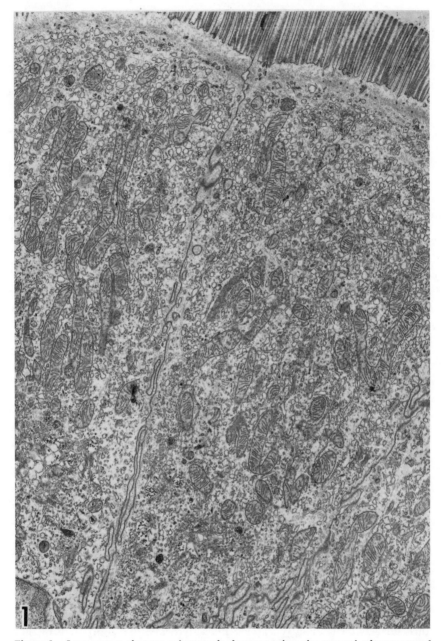

**Figure 1.** Low power electron micrograph demonstrating the general ultrastructural features of rat jejunal epithelial cells in the fasting state (×11,730).

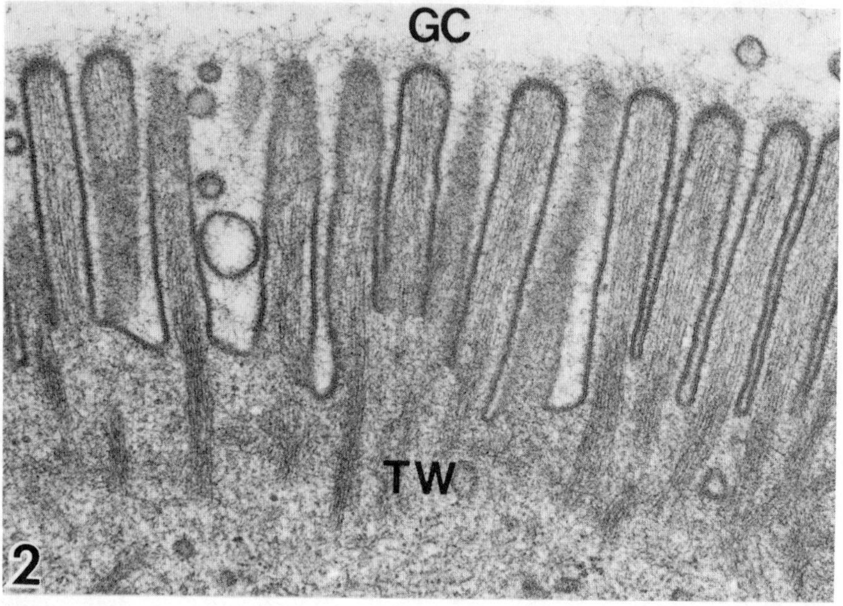

**Figure 2.** Microvilli on the surface of an intestinal absorptive cell. Note the fuzzy glycocalycx (CG) and the fibrils in the microvillus core which extend into the terminal web (TW) region (×47,430).

Cell fractionation and biochemical studies have made it possible to purify and characterize the epithelial cell brush borders (microvilli) and have elegantly defined the brush borders as a digestive–absorptive structure containing enzymes required for disaccharide and protein hydrolysis as well as carrier proteins aiding the entrance of sugars and amino acids into the cytosol (12). The microvilli are approximately 0.75–1.5 $\mu$ in length and 0.1 $\mu$ in width (Figure 2). The organization of the microvillus is complex, perhaps relating to its intimate role in so many aspects of nutrient movement. The plasma membrane comprising the microvillus surface is fundamentally similar to the bilamellar plasma membranes (Figures 2 and 3) of all cells, but differs significantly from the lateral-basal plasma membrane of the villus epithelial cells in that it is somewhat wider (95–115 Å compared to 70–80 Å) and it contains a conspicuous surface coat or glycocalyx. The glycocalyx is composed of fine filamentous material which covers the microvillus surface (Figures 2 and 3). This filamentous meshwork, or so-called "fuzzy coat," is synthesized by the individual epithelial cells and is composed of glycoproteins and acid mucopolysaccharides (13). Functionally the glycocalyx may serve as

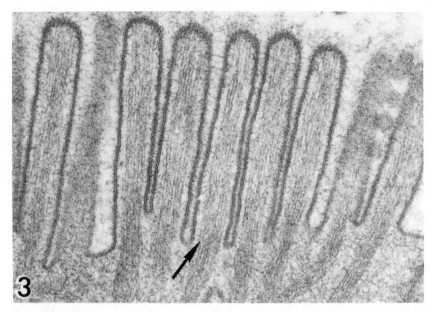

**Figure 3.** Higher magnification of intestinal microvilli showing the actin filaments glycocalyx (GC) and the fibrils in the microvillus core which extend into the terminal web where they interdigitate with myosin-containing fibrils (×72,000).

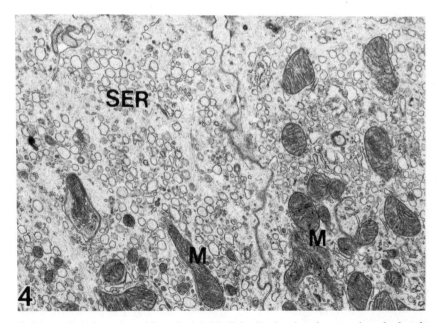

**Figure 4.** Apical portion of intestinal epithelial cells showing the smooth endoplasmic reticulum (SER) and mitochondria (×13,035).

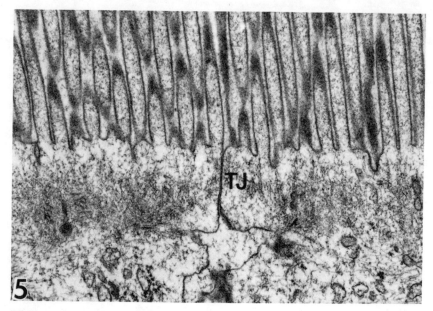

**Figure 5.**   Adjacent absorptive cells are attached by tight junctions (TJ) located in the region of the terminal web (×36,100).

a barrier against the absorption of potentially noxious substances but, more important, it is the site of localization of enzymes involved in the terminal digestion of carbohydrates and proteins. Recent studies by Weiser and collaborators (14) have shown that the glcocalyx represents, in part, the glycosolated portions of the membrane-associated enzymes including such disaccharidases as lactase and sucrase, and also peptidases and alkaline phosphatase. In very recent studies, Weiser and co-workers (15) have shown that the lateral-basal membranes of the undifferentiated crypt epithelial cells are enriched in glycosyl transferase activity, an observation that indicates a relationship between Golgi and cell surface membranes of intestinal epithelial cells.

The microvillus core is composed of a tightly packed array of filamentous structures now known to consist of actin (Figures 2 and 3). It has been proposed that the actin core of the microvilli interact with myosin-containing filaments in the terminal web region of the apical portion of the epithelial cells (16). Ultrastructural studies reveal a complex meshwork of filaments connecting the microvillus cores with the terminal web filaments (Figure 2). Exciting recent observations by Mooseker and co-workers (16, 17) have shown that the microvillus core

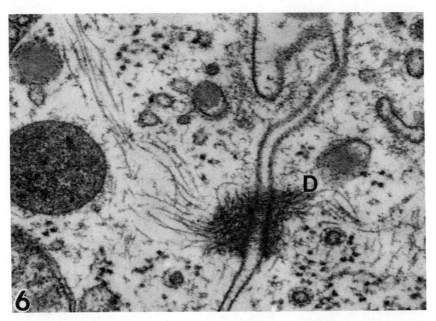

**Figure 6.** Electron micrograph illustrating the ultrastructure of a spot desmosome (D) which binds the lateral cell membranes of adjacent epithelial cells (×69,540).

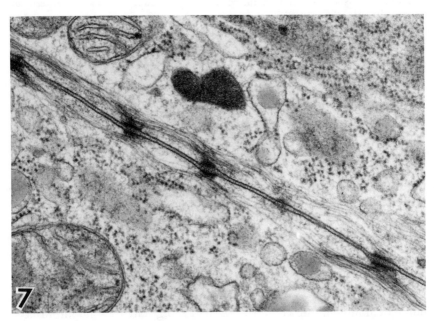

**Figure 7.** Several spot desmosomes are illustrated in this electron micrograph. Note the complex fibrilar attachments which extend into the adjacent cytosol (×41,310).

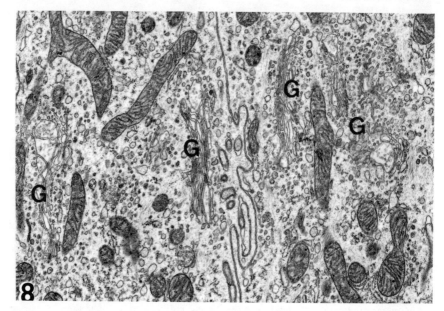

**Figure 8.** The Golgi zones (G) of two intestinal absorptive cells have a characteristic ultrastructure. Note the complex interdigitation of plasma membranes between adjacent epithelial cells (×13,825).

is composed of actin filaments and that myosin is located in the terminal web. Using isolated brush borders and polyacrylamide gel electrophoretic techniques, Mooseker and co-workers (16) have defined the properties of the brush border myosin and have shown that the positioning of actin filament–membrane attachments is optimal in respect to a polarity which would allow the actin filaments to interact with myosin to produce microvillar movements. A precise geometric location is required if anisotrophic movements are to occur. In this regard, the characterization of brush border myosin revealed physical and enzymatic properties similar to those of other vertebrate, nonmuscle myosins (16). These intriguing observations provide a biochemical and morphological basis for understanding microvillar movement.

The apical portion of the intestinal epithelial cells contains the usual complement of subcellular organelles found in most mammalian cells (Figures 1 and 4). In this regard the absorptive epithelium is not particularly specialized, containing elements of smooth and rough endoplasmic reticulum and mitochondria. In the fasting state the smooth-surfaced vesicular components are not particularly prominent (Figure 4) but, as

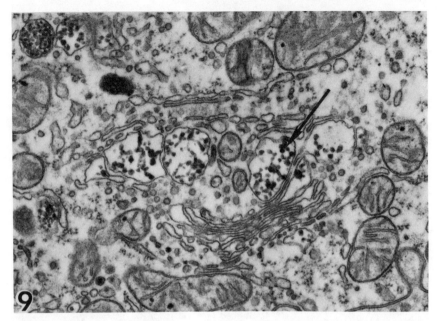

**Figure 9.** Higher power electron micrograph illustrating the ultrastructure of a Golgi apparatus in a fasting intestinal absorptive cell. Lipoprotein particles (arrow) are present in Golgi cisternae and vesicles. These represent the synthesis of endogenous VLDL by the intestinal epithelial cells (×33,840).

will be seen later, during the process of active fat absorption the smooth endoplasmic reticulum readily vesiculates as the absorbed lipolytic products accumulate within its cisternae. The intestinal epithelium is not particularly active in protein synthesis and this may be implied indirectly by the observation that the rough endoplasmic reticulum is not as extensively developed as it is, for example, in pancreatic acinar cells in which pancreatic enzyme synthesis occurs.

In fasting cells the lateral plasma membranes of adjacent epithelial cells form complex interdigitations (Figures 1 and 4) and the intracellular space is relatively insignificant (Figure 1). During active nutrient transport, the entrance of absorbed nutrients into the intercellular space is associated with a marked distension of this space, a process most vividly visualized, as will be seen later, during active lipid absorption. In recent years newer ultrastructural techniques have served to define the various junctional complexes which provide a mechanism for the adherence of cells to each other and also provide structural devices which prevent the leakage of nutrients and ions but allow cell to cell communi-

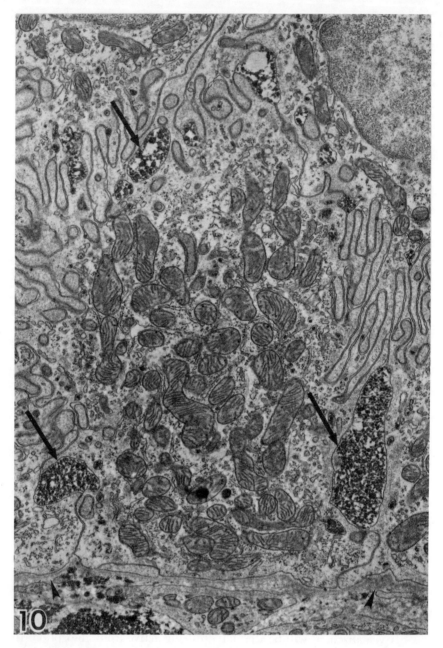

**Figure 10.** Basilar portions of several adjacent epithelial cells. Note that even in the fasting cells the intercellular spaces can be distended (arrows) by endogenously formed VLDL. The poles of the epithelial cells are separated from the lamina propria by a basement membrane (arrowheads) (×19,600).

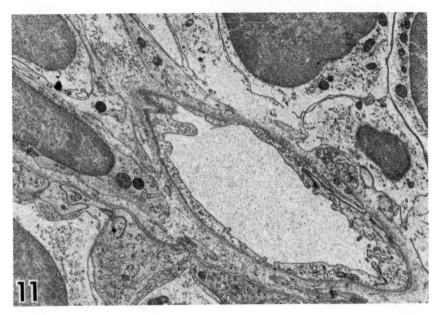

**Figure 11.** Electron micrograph showing the cellular components of the lamia propria. Seen also is a cross section of a capillary (×7,900).

cation. Junctional complexes have been described in most tissues but have been beautifully adapted to the specific transport processes of the intestinal epithelium. So-called "tight" junctions form impermeable barriers at the apical portion of adjacent epithelial cells in the region of the terminal web (Figure 5). The tight junction appears to be formed by the complete fusion of adjacent lateral plasma membranes. This fusion obliterates the intercellular space and forms an encircling belt that provides an impermeable barrier to the egress of nutrients contained within the intercellular space (18). Freeze fracture studies of the intestinal epithelium have revealed a complex organization of filaments which course through the terminal web region providing so-called "sealing strands," which bridge the opposing lateral membranes to form the tight junction complex in a manner somewhat analogous to a zipper closure (18). Also binding adjacent epithelial cells are two types of desmosomes. The belt desmosome is located near the tight junction and, as the name implies, is made up of protein fibrils which occupy the intercellular space between adjacent lateral membranes and are so organized as to completely encircle the cells, thus adding to the syncytial characteristics of the epithelium. The spot desmosomes (Figures 6 and 7) have been compared to

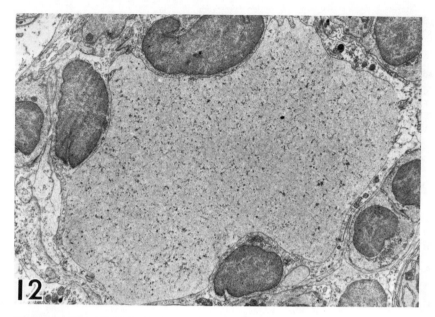

Figure 12.  Lymphatics in the lamina propria. (×5,070).

"spot welds" in character. They are composed of areas of electron-dense fibrils in the intercellular spaces, which communicate with an elaborate array of tonofilaments, which extend into the surrounding cytosol (Figures 6 and 7).

The intestinal epithelium also contains another junctional complex, termed a "gap" junction, which connects the exterior membranes of adjacent cells but at the same time permits passage of molecules from cell to cell through connecting channels of some 15 Å in greatest width (18). For example, this size is sufficient to permit passage of molecules of the size of sucrose from cell to cell. Freeze fracture studies have shown that the gap junction is formed by a mosaic of cylindrical particles.

Cells that are involved in secretion are characterized by well-defined Golgi complexes, which apparently are the site of the final assembly of secretory proteins and also generate the secretory vesicles that carry nascent particles to the surface for secretion. Prominent in this regard is the role of the intestine in fat absorption, which involves the synthesis of chylomicrons and their secretion into the intercellular space (19). In fasting cells Golgi complexes can be visualized (Figures 8 and 9), since the intestine undoubtedly synthesizes and secretes other proteins, and it is also known that endogenous very low density lipoprotein (VLDL) for-

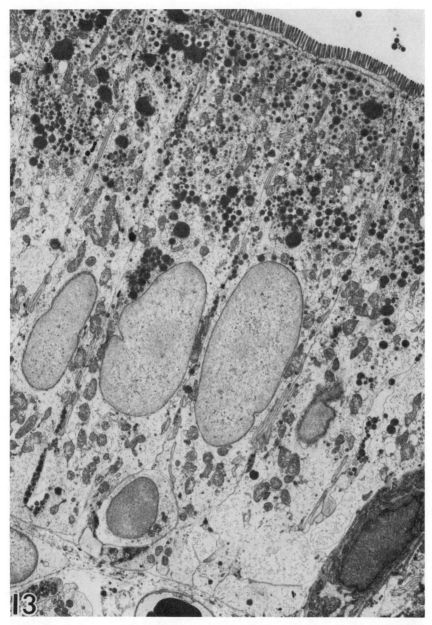

**Figure 13.** Figures 13–21 all illustrate features of fat absorption in rat jejunal epithelial cells 2 hours after feeding 1.5 ml of corn oil by gastric tube. The apical portions of jejunal absorptive cells are filled with osmiophilic lipid droplets (×3,712).

15

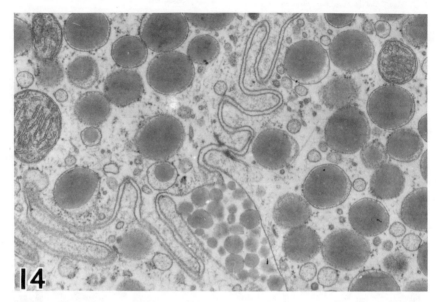

**Figure 14.** Higher power electron micrograph illustrating the accumulation of absorbed lipid within vesiculated smooth endoplasmic reticulm (×23,870).

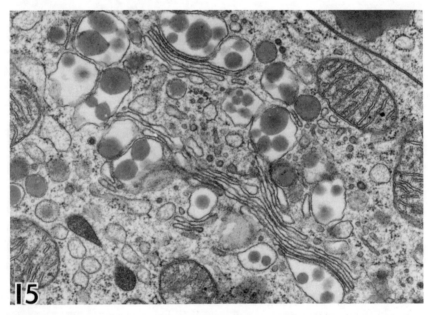

**Figure 15.** The Golgi apparatus is filled with nascent chylomicrons. Note the distention of Golgi cisternae and vesicles with chylomicron-size particles (×27,080).

16

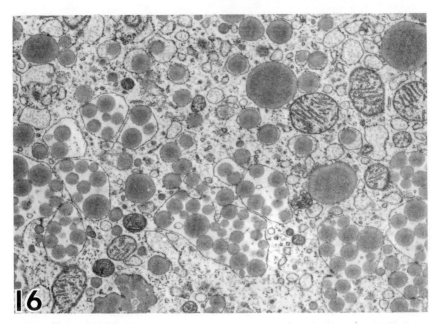

**Figure 16.** Secretory vesicles formed from the Golgi complex contain variable numbers of chylomicrons (×12,350).

mation occurs in the intestinal epithelial cells in the absence of dietary lipid (Figure 9). The Golgi complexes are characterized by parallel arrays of flattened tubular structures and vesicles frequently filled with VLDL-size particles (Figure 9). The process of endogenous VLDL formation can also be visualized by the occasional occurrence of large numbers of VLDL-size particles dilating the intercellular spaces of intestinal epithelium obtained from fasted animals (Figure 10). In these instances the intercellular spaces are distended with VLDL and the Golgi apparatus appears active in that its cisternae and vesicles are filled with VLDL.

The basal portions of the intestinal epithelial cells are applied to a basement membrane measuring approximately 300 Å wide (Figure 10). The basement membrane contains a rather homogenous material which separates the basal pole of the epithelial cells from the underlying lamina propria (Figure 10). Absorbed nutrients must cross the basal membrane and the basement membrane to enter the lamina propria, from which site entry into vascular structures or lymphatics occurs. The lamina propria (Figure 11) contains a heterogenous cellular population including plasma cells, lymphocytes, eosinophils, and mast cells. In addition, smooth muscle cells, collagen fibers, and unmyelinated nerve fibers can be found.

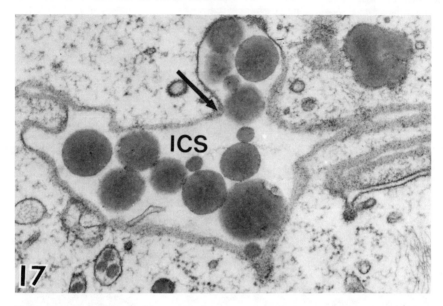

**Figure 17.** A secretory vesicle (arrow) has merged with the lateral plasma membrane of an intestinal epithelial cell and is delivering chylomicrons into the intercellular space (ICS) by the process of exocytosis (×40,260).

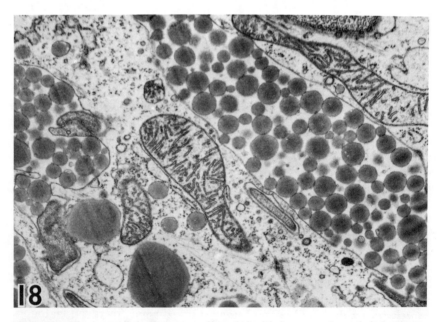

**Figure 18.** The intercellular spaces are distended with large numbers of chylomicrons in those cells which are actively absorbing fat (×17,820).

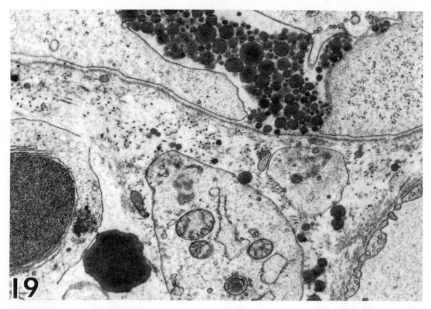

**Figure 19.** Chylomicrons in the dilated intercellular space are seen adjacent to the basement membrane. The basement membrane separates the basal portion of the epithelial cells from the lamina propria. Chylomicrons must pass through the basement membrane to enter the lamina propria (×17,400).

Of most importance for the process of nutrient absorption is the rich vascular (Figure 11) and lymphatic supply (Figure 12) of the lamina propria, which provides a ready means of access of absorbed nutrients into the vascular lymphatic system. Absorbed nutrients may enter the lumina of blood capillaries or lymphatics by diffusion across the endothelial barrier lining these structures or, as will be seen for fat absorption, by entering between gaps that open between the attenuated extensions of the endothelial cells.

## ULTRASTRUCTURAL STUDIES OF INTESTINAL LIPID ABSORPTION

The electron density of long-chain fatty acids, when they are fixed with osmium tetroxide, provides an opportunity to visualize vividly the various steps in the lipid absorptive process. Biochemical studies of intraluminal lipid digestion and intestinal absorption have defined many of the processes involved in the uptake and transport by the intestine of

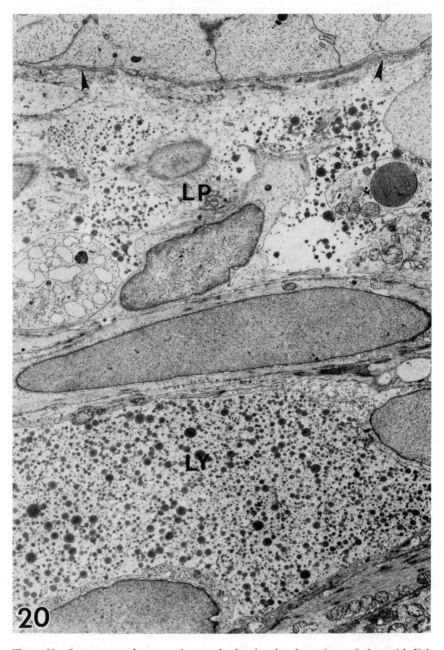

**Figure 20.** Low power electron micrograph showing basal portions of the epithelial cells (top), the basement membrane (arrowheads), chylomicrons in the lamina propria (LP), and a dilated lymphatic (LY) filled with chylomicrons (×6,650).

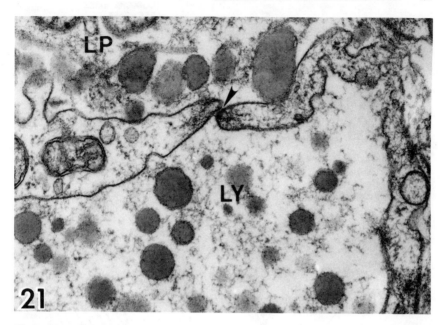

**Figure 21.** The arrowhead points to a junction between the endothelial cells lining a lymphatic (LY). Chylomicrons filter from the lamina propria (LP) into the lymphatic through these endothelial junctions (×44,370).

dietary lipid (20). The biochemical aspects of lipid absorption are described in Chapter 2. This section will deal only with the ultrastructural features of the assembly, intracellular transport, and secretion of chylomicrons, thereby providing an opportunity to describe the role of intracellular organelles in the absorption of one type of nutrient. Figures 13–21 are sequential illustrations of lipid absorption in rats fed 1.5 ml of corn oil by stomach tube. Although all of the electron micrographs were taken in biopsies removed 2 hours after corn oil feeding, similar images can be found at earlier or later times, 2 hours being selected as a convenient time in which a composite picture of the various phases of fat absorption can be illustrated easily.

The major products of intraluminal triglyceride digestion (fatty acids, monoglycerides) are transported into the absorptive cells by passive diffusion from bile salt micellar solutions (21). Although earlier studies (22) suggested uptake by pinocytosis, the latter process has been effectively ruled out and there is now little controversy concerning the rapid penetration of lipolytic products into the cell by diffusion through the plasma membrane of the microvillus surface. As visualized by the electron micro-

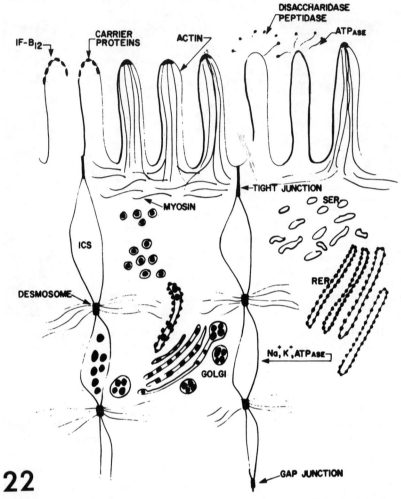

**22**

**Figure 22.** Diagrammatic representation of an intestinal epithelial cell depicting the localization of digestive enzymes, specific transport proteins and enzymes, and subcellular structures that are involved in nutrient movement.

scope the first phase of absorption consists of the appearance of innumerable osmiophilic droplets in the apical portion of the cells just beneath the terminal web region (Figure 13). These droplets, representing the absorbed lipolytic products, are contained within vesiculated elements of the smooth endoplasmic reticulum (Figure 14). The juxtaposition of the lipolytic products to the membranes of the smooth endoplasmic reticulum appears to be more than fortuitous, since the latter are known to contain the enzyme systems responsible for triglyceride esterification. Electron microscopy cannot discriminate between the chemical form of the absorbed lipid; therefore, one can only infer that droplets appearing in the most apical region represent the still untransformed absorbed lipolytic products. The vesicular appearance of the smooth endoplasmic reticulum represents cross-sectioned profiles of the hyperplastic endoplasmic reticulum which seems to form rapidly in response to fat absorption. In the supranuclear region of the cell the Golgi complexes (Figure 15) become filled with chylomicron-size particles which distend the Golgi cisternae and vesicles. As indicated earlier, Golgi complexes can be visualized in fasting cells and may contain endogenous VLDL; however, there is a striking proliferation of Golgi elements during the active phase of fat absorption and Golgi complexes become enlarged secondary to distension with chylomicrons and proliferation of cisternal and vesicular components (Figure 15).

Examination of many electron micrographs provides the impression of an intracellular transport of absorbed lipid through elements of smooth and rough endoplasmic reticulum and thence to the Golgi complex. Current concepts suggest the formation of smooth endoplasmic reticulum from the rough endoplasmic reticulum, and there is some evidence that the apoprotein moieties of the chylomicrons are added to the newly formed triglycerides at the junction between rough and smooth endoplasmic reticulum. Direct structural continuities between the endoplasmic reticulum and the Golgi zones have not been visualized. It would appear that vesicles containing nascent chylomicrons, formed from the endoplasmic reticulum, migrate to the Golgi zone and merge with Golgi components, thereby bringing the nascent chylomicrons to the site where the final assembly of the chylomicrons occurs prior to secretion (19).

The accumulation of nascent chylomicrons in the Golgi complex stimulates the formation of secretory vesicles, which are directly derived from Golgi components (Figure 16). The secretory vesicles, containing variable numbers of chylomicrons, migrate through the cytoplasm toward the lateral plasma membrane. There is apparently some specificity of recognition between the secretory vesicle membrane and the lateral plasma membrane but the chemical nature of this presumed recognition site is

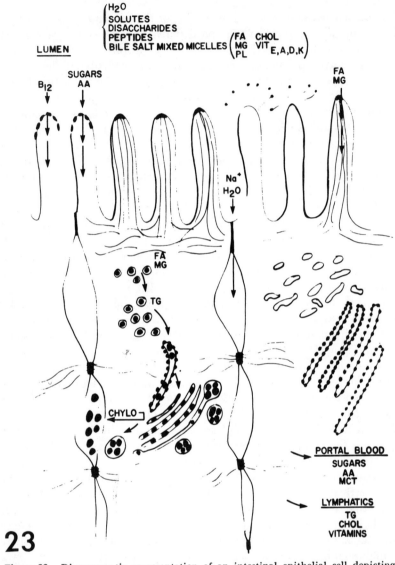

**Figure 23.** Diagrammatic representation of an intestinal epithelial cell depicting the sites and pathways of nutrient absorption (AA, amino acids; FA, fatty acids; MG, monoglycerides; PL, phospholipids; TG, triglycerides; chol, cholesterol; MCT, medium-chain triglycerides.)

not known. In any event the secretory vesicle membrane fuses with the lateral plasmalemma, and thus discharges its content of chylomicrons into the intercellular space (Figure 17). The intercellular spaces become distended with innumerable chylomicrons (Figure 18), which find their way to the basal poles of the epithelial cells (Figure 19), where they must then cross the basal membrane and the basement membrane separating the epithelium from the lamina propria (Figure 19). Some electron microscopic images suggest that chylomicrons enter the lamina propria by passing through gaps in the basement membranes; however, it is frequently difficult to visualize such gaps and many electron micrographs illustrate chylomicrons on either side of an intact basement membrane (Figure 19). Following entrance into the lamina propria the chylomicrons percolate through the cellular constituents of the lamina propria (Figure 20) and eventually find their way into the lymphatics, which are entered through gaps between adjacent endothelial cells (Figure 21). In nonabsorbing cells the fingerlike extensions of the endothelial cells overlap and form a continuous lining; however, during active fat absorption, gaps between endothelial cells are frequently visualized and this would appear to form a mechanism for chylomicron entry into the lymphatics (Figure 21).

This somewhat abbreviated description of intestinal fat absorption highlights the major points that can be visualized by electron microscopy of actively absorbing intestinal epithelial cells. Of major importance is the step by step translocation of nascent chylomicrons through the various subcellular compartments during which time many biochemical processes occur, resulting in the resynthesis of triglycerides and the formation of chylomicrons. Essential in this regard is passage through the Golgi apparatus, where the final assembly or synthesis of the nascent chylomicron occurs (19). Since the Golgi complex is active in glycosolation reactions it is possible that the final aspect of chylomicron biosynthesis involves the glycosolation of incomplete glycoproteins, a process which may be required for secretory vesicle formation.

This chapter has briefly reviewed the ultrastructural organization of the intestinal epithelium, emphasizing those aspects of cellular structure which are involved in the unidirectional flow of nutrients from the intestinal lumen into the cell, and from there into the intercellular spaces and vascular or lymphatic systems. As seen in Figure 22, the intestinal epithelium is exquisitely differentiated in regard to its structural and chemical composition, thereby permitting the unidirectional absorption of specific nutrients. This differentiation includes, at the luminal surface, a digestive–absorptive surface with an enormous surface area containing enzymes required for the terminal digestion of carbohydrates and proteins, a plasma membrane containing carrier proteins required for nutrient transport into the cytoplasm, and even receptors which define the molecular basis for the absorption of vitamin $B_{12}$. The lateral plasma membrane contains $Na^+$, $K^+$, ATPase, thus providing a mechanism for the transport of solutes across the lateral cell membrane into the intercellular spaces, while the presence of junctional complexes provides a means for cell to cell communication but prevents the loss of nutrients by "leaking" from the intercellular spaces back into the intestinal lumen. The organelles which comprise the intracellular compartment contain enzyme systems required for triglyceride, phospholipid, and cholesterol synthesis, and specific proteins such as chylomicron and VLDL apoproteins (e.g., apoB, apoA-I) can be synthesized by the rough endoplasmic reticulum (Figure 23). The secretory pathway for chylomicrons is aided by active Golgi complexes which complete the assembly of nascent chylomicrons prior to secretion. The biochemical and molecular events involved in nutrient absorption (Figure 23) will be the subject of other chapters. I hope that this review has provided an appropriate morphological basis for understanding the complex events involved in the transport of each specific class of nutrient.

## REFERENCES

1. G. G. Forstner, S. M. Sabesin, and K. J. Isselbacher, *Biochem. J.*, **106**, 381 (1968).

2. U. Hopper, K. Nelson, J. Perrotto, and K. J. Isselbacher, *J. Biol. Chem.*, **248**, 25 (1973).

3. J. S. Trier and C. E. Rubin, *Gastroenterology*, **40**, 574 (1965).

4. L. A. Staehelin, *Int. Rev. Cytol.*, **39**, 191 (1974).

5. A. Eichholz and R. K. Crane, *J. Cell Biol.*, **26**, 687 (1965).

6. J. P. Quigley and G. S. Gotterer, *Biochim. Biophys. Acta*, **173**, 456 (1969).

7. M. Fujita, H. Ohta, K. Kawai, H. Matsui, and M. Nakao, *Biochim. Biophys. Acta*, **274**, 336 (1972).

8. R. R. Cardell, Jr., S. Badenhausen, and K. Porter, *J. Cell Biol.*, **34**, 123 (1967).

9. E. W. Strauss, in C. F. Code, Ed., *Handbook of Physiology*, American Physiological Society, Washington, D.C., 1966, p. 1377.

10. J. S. Trier, *Fed. Proc.*, **26**, 139 (1967).

11. H. I. Friedman and R. R. Cardell, Jr., *J. Cell Biol.*, **52**, 15 (1972).

12. R. K. Crane, in W. Heidel, Ed., *Handbook of Physiology*, Vol. III, American Physiological Society, Washington, D.C., 1968, p. 1323.

13. S. Ito, *Fed. Proc.*, **28**, 12 (1969).

14. M. M. Weiser, *J. Biol. Chem.*, **248**, 2542 (1973).

15. M. M. Weiser, M. M. Neumeier, A. Quaroni, and K. Kirsch, *J. Cell Biol.*, **77**, 722 (1978).

16. M. S. Mooseker and L. G. Tilney, *J. Cell Biol.,* **67,** 725 (1975).
17. M. S. Mooseker, T. D. Pollard, and K. Fujiwara, *J. Cell Biol.,* **79,** 444 (1978).
18. B. E. Hull and L. A. Staehelin, *J. Cell Biol.,* **68,** 688 (1976).
19. S. M. Sabesin and S. Frase, *J. Lipid Res.,* **18,** 496 (1977).
20. J. R. Senior, *J. Lipid Res.,* **5,** 495 (1964).
21. E. W. Strauss, *J. Lipid Res.,* **7,** 307 (1966).
22. S. L. Palay and L. J. Karlin, *J. Biophys. Biochem. Cytol.,* **5,** 373 (1959).

# 2

## Intestinal Fat Absorption

ROBERT M. GLICKMAN, M.D.

College of Physicians and Surgeons, Columbia University, New York, New York

The average western diet contains approximately 40% of total calories as dietary fat, or approximately 100 g/day of fat. Fat absorption is a multistep process, involving the coordinated participation of several organs (Figure 1). The efficiency of the entire process can be judged by the fact that under normal conditions less than 5% of ingested fat is recovered in the stool. Since the process may become deranged at any step, an understanding of factors important in fat absorption will facilitate the understanding of clinical conditions of fat malabsorption.

As shown in Figure 1 the overall process of fat absorption can be conveniently considered to be composed of (*a*) luminal, (*b*) mucosal, and (*c*) secretory (lymphatic or portal) transport. This chapter is not intended to be an exhaustive review of the subject but rather will stress the newer information that has become available.

### INTRALUMINAL DIGESTION

Most dietary fat is ingested in the form of triglycerides containing three long-chain fatty acids on a glycerol backbone. Triglycerides are insoluble in the aqueous environment of the intestinal lumen and hence form an oily interface with water. Such large oil droplets cannot be taken up into the intestinal epithelial cell in this form. Rather, triglycerides are acted upon by triglyceride lipases which split off the two fatty acids at the end of the molecule, leaving a single fatty acid combined with the glycerol as a monoglyceride. Although lingual and gastric lipases have been described, it is the pancreatic lipase that is responsible for most triglyceride

**29**

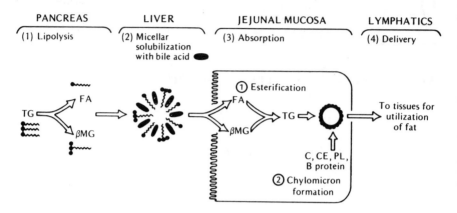

**Figure 1.** Schematic representation of intestinal fat absorption showing the participation of pancreas, liver, and intestinal mucosal cell in fat absorption [Wilson and Dietschy (8)].

hydrolysis. Recent information has shown that for pancreatic lipase to be active in triglyceride hydrolysis an additional pancreatic factor is required. This factor is a small molecular weight protein ($\sim$ 10,000) secreted by the pancreas and called colipase (1). Colipase facilitates lipase action by binding to bile salt–lipid surfaces and facilitates the interaction of lipase with triglyceride, permitting efficient hydrolysis. Other requirements for efficient lipolysis are an intraluminal pH greater than 4, and bile salts which are required for optimal lipase action. In addition, pancreatic secretion must be closely coordinated with the presence of lipid in the upper intestine. This is accomplished by the effect of lipid and protein-releasing cholecystokinin-pancreozymin (CCK-PZ) from intestinal epithelial cells in the duodenum, with resultant stimulation of pancreatic enzyme secretion. The CCK-PZ also causes gallbladder contraction and relaxation of the sphincter of Oddi to enable bile salt secretion to be synchronous with the presence of fat in the upper intestine.

Similarly, gastric acid releases secretin from duodenal mucosa, which stimulates pancreatic fluid and bicarbonate secretion, an important factor in raising duodenal pH to permit effective lipolysis.

With these considerations in mind, clinical disorders leading to impaired lipolysis can be more easily understood (Table 1) (8).

The products of triglyceride lipolysis, although more water soluble than the parent triglyceride, still have only limited solubility in the aqueous environment of the intestinal lumen. This is also true for lipids such as cholesterol and fat-soluble vitamins such as vitamins A, D, E, and K. Efficient absorption depends on the process of micelle formation in which

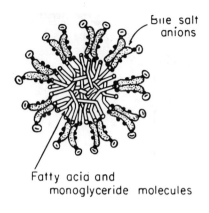 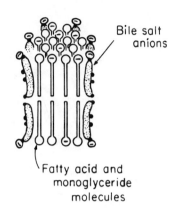

**Figure 2.** Schematic representation of fatty acid, monglyceride bile salt micelle. In both representations the bile salts surround the less polar lipid moieties.

lipid moieties such as fatty acids, monoglycerides, and cholesterol interact with bile salts in mixed aggregates or micelles. A schematic representation of a bile salt micelle containing fatty acids, monoglycerides, and bile salts is shown in Figure 2.

It is the particular structural characteristics of the bile salt molecule, consisting of hydrophobic and hydrophilic portions, which enables these amphipathic molecules to interact with lipids in an aqueous environment and solubilize these moieties (2–4). Conjugation of the bile acids with

**Table 1    Conditions Associated with Impaired Lipolysis**

1. Postgastrectomy
    a. Rapid transit
    b. Improper mixing of triglyceride with pancreatic lipase, i.e., Billroth Type 2 anastomosis
2. Altered duodenal pH
    a. Acid hypersecretion (Zollinger Ellison syndrome)
3. Decreased CCK-PZ release
    Severe intestinal mucosal destruction, i.e., sprue
4. Pancreatic insufficiency → ↓ lipase, ↓ bicarbonate (7)
    a. Chronic pancreatitis
    b. Obstruction of pancreatic duct
5. Decreased luminal bile salts
    Multiple causes—see Table 2

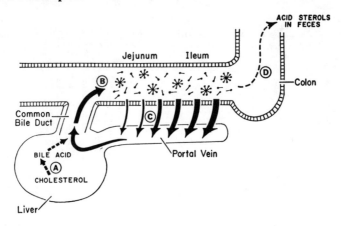

**Figure 3.** Schematic representation of the enterohepatic circulation of bile salts.

either glycine or taurine further improves their detergent properties at the pH of the upper intestine. As schematically shown in Figure 3, bile acids are formed from cholesterol in the liver and enter the upper intestine to participate in micelle formation. Although maximal absorption of lipid takes place in the upper small intestine, only minor absorption of bile salts occurs at this location. Rather, there is a specific active transport system in the terminal ileum that is responsible for active bile salt absorption. The efficiency of this distal absorptive mechanism is apparent when one considers that approximately 20–30 g of bile salts enter the intestine daily and only 500 mg of bile salts are lost in the stool. This

### Table 2   Conditions Associated with Impaired Micelle Formation

1. Decreased hepatic synthesis of bile salts
   Severe parenchymal liver disease
2. Decreased delivery of bile salts to the intestinal lumen
   Biliary obstruction (stone, tumor)
3. Increased intestinal loss of bile salts
   Ileal resection of disease (regional enteritis)
4. Alterations of bile salts within the intestinal lumen
   Increased acidity (Zollinger Ellison)—decreased ionization
   of bile salts with increased proximal absorption
   Precipitation of bile salts—drugs such as neomycin,
   cholestyramine

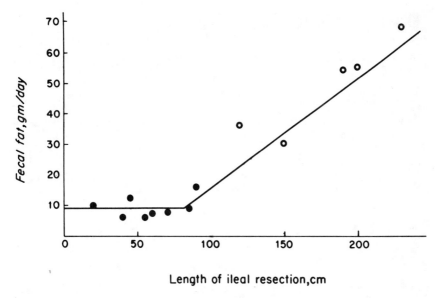

**Figure 4.** Relation between length of ileal resection, and degree of steatorrhea [Hofmann and Poley (6)].

daily loss of bile salts is matched by an approximately equal synthesis by the liver. It is this enterohepatic circulation of bile acids that permits reutilization of a limited bile acid pool (2–4 g) approximately 8–10 times daily. To accommodate the needs of lipid absorption, the bile acid pool may be recycled several times during the course of a single meal. From this brief overview of bile salt metabolism, one can predict the conditions that will result in a decreased concentration of bile salts within the intestinal lumen (below the critical micellar concentration) and result in impaired micellar solubilization of lipids (Table 2).

A particularly graphic example of impaired micelle formation leading to steatorrhea is that associated with ileal resection (5, 6). As shown in Figure 4, with modest degrees of ileal resection (less than 100 cm), increased hepatic synthesis of bile salts can compensate for the increased fecal loss, maintaining the micellar concentration of bile acids in the jejunum within normal limits. Thus there is no resultant steatorrhea. With larger degrees of ileal resection (greater than 100 cm), hepatic synthesis is maximally increased but cannot compensate for these large fecal losses. Therefore jejunal bile acid concentrations fall, and steatorrhea results. In this clinical situation lipolysis and mucosal epithelial function are normal and the malabsorption is a "pure" example of bile salt deficiency. This

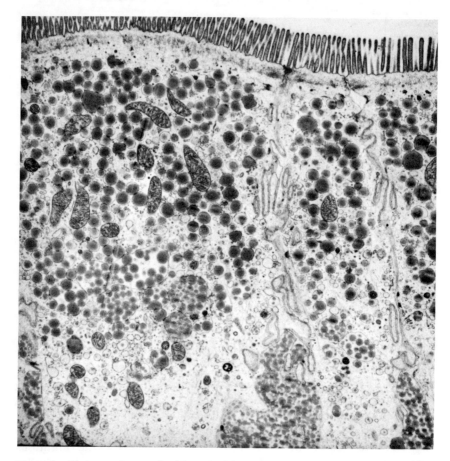

**Figure 5.**   Electron micrograph of intestinal fat absorption. Droplets of triglyceride are first visible within the profiles of the smooth endoplasmic reticulum beneath the microvillus membrane. The entire apical portion of the cell contains lipid droplets and chylomicrons are abundant in the lateral intercellular spaces.

disorder also underscores the obligatory requirement of active ileal bile salt absorption, a function that cannot be assumed by the more proximal small bowel.

## MUCOSAL PHASE OF FAT ABSORPTION

Successful micellarization of lipids within the intestinal lumen permits these lipid products to diffuse to the surface of the intestinal epithelium and make intimate contact with the microvillus membrane. This is par-

ticularly important since it has been shown experimentally that surrounding the surface of the intestine is an unstirred water layer which
functionally may pose a significant barrier to the diffusion of hydrophobic molecules, such as lipids. This relatively immobile aqueous layer is
more easily penetrated by the micellar complex, thus increasing the efficiency of lipid uptake into the intestinal mucosal cell.

The uptake of lipids such as fatty acids and monoglycerides across the
microvillus membrane is a passive process and results from the solubility
of the lipid moieties within the lipid-rich surface membrane of the epithelial cell. Recently, a low molecular weight cytosolic protein, fatty acid
binding protein (FABP), has been isolated from the intestine (10). This
protein avidly binds fatty acids and appears to function as an intracellular transport protein for long-chain fatty acids. Under experimental conditions where fatty acid binding to this protein is inhibited, less fatty
acid is available for triglyceride resynthesis. Thus it appears that FABP
may serve a transport function within the intestinal epithelium to direct
intracellular fatty acids to the smooth endoplasmic reticulum, the site of
triglyceride resynthesis. One may wonder why, after the luminal hydrolysis of dietary triglycerides and their uptake into the cell, triglyceride
resynthesis is necessary. It is probable that such a mechanism reduces the
effective concentration of free fatty acids within the cell and maintains
an effective concentration gradient for passive uptake to continue. In
addition, the storage of fatty acids as the more inert triglycerides while
awaiting transport from the intestine may spare the cell the potential
injurious effects of high free fatty acid concentrations.

The enzymes for triglyceride resynthesis have been localized biochemi-
cally to the smooth endoplasmic reticulum in the apical portion of the
intestinal epithelial cell beneath the microvillus membrane. This is cor-
roborated morphologically in that triglyceride is first visualized within
the intestinal epithelial cell within the profiles of the smooth endoplasmic reticulum (Figure 5). As shown in this figure, shortly after lipid
absorption, the entire apical portion of the intestinal cell is filled with
triglyceride droplets. Morphologically, one can follow the movement with
time of these triglyceride droplets through the profiles of the endoplasmic
reticulum to the Golgi apparatus in the supranuclear portion of the cell.
Here clusters of chylomicrons can be seen within the saccules of the
Golgi apparatus. Although few details are known about the actual mechanisms of lipoprotein egress from the cell, morphological studies show a
migration of Golgi vesicles toward the lateral-basal aspect of the cell.
These Golgi vesicles then appear to fuse with the plasma membrane in
this location and discharge their contents into the intercellular space by
reverse pinocytosis. It has been suggested that this directed intracellular

Table 3   Characteristics of Rat Intestinal
Lymph Chylomicrons

| Chemical Composition | (%) |
|---|---|
| Triglyceride | 84 |
| Phospholipid | 13 |
| Cholesterol | 2 |
| Protein | 1 |
| Density | <1.006 g/ml |
| $S_f$ value | >400 |
| Electrophoresis | origin |

movement of triglyceride may depend in part on intact microtubular function.

Although the morphologic events of triglyceride transport have been well defined, less is known about the biochemical events of chylomicron formation. A great deal can be learned by analyzing the composition of chylomicrons obtained from mesenteric lymph of laboratory animals or thoracic duct lymph of man. Table 3 shows the chemical composition of rat intestinal lymph chylomicrons.

It is apparent that triglyceride makes up the major portion of chylomicron lipid, which is in keeping with the major physiological role of this particle in fat absorption. Phospholipid, although quantitatively smaller, is important structurally. Together with chylomicron protein and free cholesterol, chylomicron phospholipid is arranged on the surface of this spherical particle. Although the intestine can synthesize phospholipid de novo for the chylomicron surface, normally a large proportion of chylomicron phospholipid is derived from luminal phospholipid (i.e., biliary lecithin) after reacylation of absorbed lysolecithin. Similarly, the cholesterol of chylomicrons is derived from dietary and luminal sources, with approximately 50–75% esterified within the mucosal cell before being secreted in the form of chylomicrons.

The protein of the chylomicrons has been the subject of considerable interest. Although quantitatively small (1% of chylomicron mass), chylomicron apoproteins contain a characteristic complement of specific proteins. Figure 6 shows the apoprotein composition of rat and human lymph chylomicrons after delipidation and electrophoresis on SDS acrylamide gels. It can be seen that there is a remarkable similarity in the protein patterns from these two species. Most of the proteins have been well identified and characterized and their names have been indicated. Of particular importance to intestinal lipid transport is apoB as discussed below. In addition, apoA-I, the major apoprotein of circulating high

CHYLOMICRON
APOPROTEINS

RAT      HUMAN

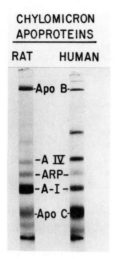

**Figure 6.** Apoprotein composition of rat mesenteric lymph and human chylomicrons (isolated from chyluria). The aproproteins are separated on sodium dodecyl sulfate polyacrylamide gels.

density lipoproteins in most species, is also an important chylomicron component and makes up 20% of chylomicron protein in man and 40% in the rat. A newly described chylomicron apoprotein in man, apoA-IV, is analogous to a similar apoprotein in the rat. Its metabolic importance remains to be determined. A group of small molecular weight apoproteins, the C apoproteins, are also characteristically found on lymph chylomicrons. One of this group, apoC-II, is an activator of lipoprotein lipase and therefore is extremely important in the catabolism of chylomicrons after secretion.

Since lymph is an ultrafiltrate of plasma and apoproteins have been shown to exchange among plasma lipoproteins, one cannot be certain that a given apoprotein, despite being associated with lymph chylomicrons, originates in the intestine. It is therefore necessary to determine which of these apoproteins is actively synthesized by the intestinal mucosal cell during chylomicron formation. Experimentally, one approach to this problem is to observe the incorporation of radioactive amino acids into the various chylomicron apoproteins of lymph during lipid absorption in the rat. As shown in Figure 7, only three chylomicron apoproteins appear to be de novo synthesized during chylomicron formation —apoB, apoA-IV, and apoA-I. The other chylomicron apoproteins are acquired by the particle after secretion by the intestinal cell via transfer from other lipoproteins.

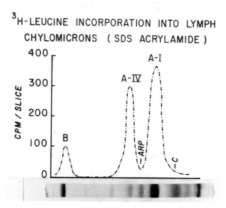

**Figure 7.** De novo synthesis of rat chylomicron apoproteins obtained from mesenteric lymph.

Although apoproteins are quantitatively a small proportion of chylomicron mass, apoprotein synthesis appears to be extremely critical for triglyceride transport through the intestinal mucosa (11, 12). Figure 8 shows an intestinal biopsy from a patient after an 18 hour fast. It can be seen that the mucosa is engorged with large droplets, which on analysis are triglyceride droplets. Such an appearance in the fasting state is abnormal and suggests an impairment in triglyceride transport. This biopsy was obtained from a patient with abetalipoproteinemia, a rare hereditary disorder associated with a total inability to form triglyceride-rich lipoproteins. Similar biopsies have been seen in human protein-calorie malnutrition (17) as well as in experimental conditions in animals with impaired protein synthesis. Thus intact protein synthesis appears to be necessary for chylomicron formation to proceed.

It has been shown in experimental animals and man that the intestinal mucosa in the fasting state contains a small pool of chylomicron apoproteins (13, 14). This pool becomes rapidly depleted during the initial stages of chylomicron formation and new apoprotein synthesis is required to permit continued chylomicron formation to proceed (15). Experimentally, once this pool is depleted and protein synthesis is impaired, triglyceride accumulates within the cell (16). Although it has not been proven, a similar defect may exist in protein-calorie malnutrition. Perhaps the most graphic example of impaired apoprotein synthesis resulting in defective intestinal triglyceride absorption is in the disease

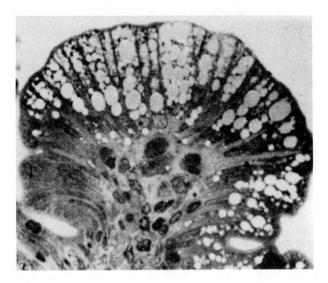

**Figure 8.** Intestinal biopsy after an 18 hour fast in a patient with abetalipoproteinemia.

abetalipoproteinemia. It has recently been shown that the intestinal mucosa of such patients, despite being engorged with triglyceride, completely lacks immunoreactive apoB. It appears that other apoproteins are normal. Thus, this rare disease has clearly shown that apoB synthesis is an obligatory step in chylomicron formation and in its absence there is a total inability to form chylomicrons. Although there are no known human disease states with an inability to synthesize apoA-I or apoA-IV, experimental studies in animals suggest that these apoproteins are not absolutely required for chylomicron formation to proceed.

Although studies of chylomicron apoprotein synthesis have not been carried out in various human malabsorptive disorders, it is probable that in mucosal destructive diseases (i.e., sprue) or severe protein-calorie malnutrition, impaired apoprotein synthesis is a contributing factor in the resultant malabsorption. In addition, it is probable that the complex series of synthetic steps required for chylomicron formation is most fully developed in mature, differentiated, villus epithelial cells. It is not known whether less differentiated cells along the villus can absorb lipid as efficiently as fully differentiated villus cells. In disease states such as sprue or during intestinal repair or regeneration functionally immature (less differentiated) epithelial cells populate the intestinal villus. Such cells may have a limited capacity for chylomicron formation; however, this remains to be proven. Similar studies are required to determine whether the decreased capacity of the distal intestine for chylomicron formation is due to a relative impairment of apoprotein synthesis.

## LIPOPROTEIN SECRETION

As stated above lymphatic transport is required for triglyceride-rich lipo-proteins to reach the systemic circulation after secretion from the intestinal cell. One would anticipate that lymphatic obstruction would impair intestinal fat transport. Such is the case in diseases associated with lymphatic obstruction, such as intestinal lymphangiectasia, Whipple's disease, and lymphoma, where lymphatic obstruction is not uncommon. In such situations the therapeutic use of medium-chain triglycerides is advantageous, since fatty acids of less than 12 carbons in length are not incorporated into chylomicrons (3). These short-chain fatty acids pass directly into the portal blood and thus provide the caloric supplementation of fat without requiring chylomicron formation or lymphatic transport.

## THE IMPORTANCE OF THE INTESTINE IN SYSTEMIC LIPOPROTEIN METABOLISM

There is mounting evidence that the intestine is a major source for the synthesis of apoprotein constituents of important plasma lipoproteins. As noted above apoproteins such as apoB, apoA-I, and apoA-IV are actively synthesized by the intestine during chylomicron formation. Since these lipoproteins of intestinal origin enter the systemic circulation, they directly contribute to the levels of these apoproteins in plasma. This is especially true for apoA-I, which has been shown to leave the chylomicron surface after secretion and eventuate in plasma high density lipoproteins. Estimates in man indicate that as much as 50% of the total daily synthesis of this apoprotein may originate in the intestine and thus directly influence plasma high density lipoprotein metabolism (18). Future research is required to determine factors which modulate the intestinal synthesis of such apoproteins. Sufficient data are already available to indicate that dietary influences and their effects on the quantitative and qualitative aspects of intestinal lipoprotein formation will have important consequences for systemic lipoprotein metabolism.

# REFERENCES

1. B. Borgstrom, On the interactions between pancreatic lipase and colipase and the substrate, and the importance of bile salts, *J. Lipid Res.*, **16,** 411 (1975).

2. R. K. Ockner and K. J. Isselbacher, Recent concepts of intestinal fat absorption, *Rev. Physiol. Biochem. Pharmacol.*, **71,** 107 (1974).

3. N. J. Greenberger and T. G. Skillman, Medium chain triglycerides. Physiological considerations and clinical implications, *New Engl. J. Med.*, **280,** 1045 (1969).

4. A. F. Hofmann, Clinical implications of physiochemical studies on bile salts, *Gastroenterology*, **48,** 484 (1965).

5. W. I. Austad, L. Lack, and M. P. Tyor, Importance of bile acids and of an intact distal small intestine for fat absorption, *Gastroenterology*, **52,** 638 (1967).

6. A. F. Hofmann and J. R. Poley, Role of bile acid malabsorption in pathogenesis of diarrhea and steatorrhea in patients with ileal resection, *Gastroenterology*, **62,** 918 (1972).

7. E. Di Magno, V. L. Go, and W. H. Summerskill, Relations between pancreatic enzyme outputs and malabsorption in severe pancreatic insufficiency, *New Engl. J. Med.*, **288,** 813 (1973).

8. F. A. Wilson and J. M. Dietschy, Differential diagnostic approach to clinical problems of malabsorption, *Gastroenterology*, **61,** 911 (1971).

9. R. R. Cardell, Jr., S. Badenhausen, and K. P. Porter, Intestinal triglyceride absorption in the rat. An electronmicroscopical study, *J. Cell Biol.*, **34,** 125 (1967).

10. R. K. Ockner and J. A. Manning, Fatty acid binding protein: Role in esterification of absorbed long chain fat in rat intestine, *J. Clin. Invest.*, **58,** 632 (1976).

11. R. I. Levy, D. S. Frederickson, and L. Laster, The lipoproteins and lipid transport in abetalipoproteinemia, *J. Clin. Invest.*, **45,** 531 (1966).

12. R. M. Glickman, Chylomicron formation by the intestine, in K. Rommel, Univ. of Ulm and H. Goebell, Univ. of Essen, Eds., *Lipid Absorption: Biochemical and Clinical Aspects*, 1975.

13. R. M. Glickman, J. Khorana, and A. Kilgore, Localization of apolipoprotein B in intestinal epithelial cells, *Science*, **193,** 1254, (1976).

14. R. M. Glickman, P. H. R. Green, R. S. Lees, S. E. Lux, and A. Kilgore, Immunofluorescence studies of apolipoprotein B in intestinal mucosa: Absence in abetalipoproteinemia, *Gastroenterology*, **76,** 288 (1979).

15. R. M. Glickman and K. Kirsch, Lymph chylomicron formation during the inhibition of protein synthesis, *J. Clin. Invest.*, 2910 (1973).

16. R. M. Glickman, A. Kilgore, and J. Khorana, Chylomicron apoprotein localization within rat intestinal epithelium: Studies of normal and impaired lipid absorption, *J. Lipid Res.*, **19,** 260 (1978).

17. J. J. Theron, W. Wittmann, J. G. Prinslou, The fine structure of the jejunum in kwashiorkor, *Exp. Mol. Path.*, **14,** 184 (1971).

18. R. M. Glickman and P. H. R. Green, The intestine as a source of apolipoprotein A-I, *PNAS*, **74,** 2569 (1977).

# 3

## Absorption and Malabsorption of Dietary Carbohydrate

GARY M. GRAY, M.D.

Stanford University School of Medicine, Stanford, California

### DIETARY CARBOHYDRATES, LUMINAL DIGESTION OF STARCH

Carbohydrate continues to be an inexpensive source of calories world-wide. The principal dietary carbohydrates are starches, sucrose, and lactose. All of these must be digested to the final monosaccharide products before they can be assimilated across the intestinal surface membrane. Starch is hydrolyzed in the intestinal lumen and its oligosaccharide products are digested by integral enzymes of the intestinal brush border. The disaccharides lactose and sucrose, rather than being altered by intraluminal enzymes, are hydrolyzed exclusively by contact with specific carbohydrases that are constituents of the intestinal surface membrane.

Starch, the principal dietary saccharide, comprising 60% of the carbohydrate calories in the western diet, is a glucose-containing polysaccharide consisting of a chain of $\alpha$ 1,4 glucosyl units and having a molecular weight of 100,000 to more than 1 million. Most starches are of the branched or amylopectin type by virtue of having about 5% $\alpha$ 1,6 branching linkages. The alpha type of linkage between adjacent glucosyl residues is crucial for specificity of the hydrolytic enzymes that are responsible for cleaving starch to the final glucose products. Thus, $\alpha$-amylase is incapable of cleaving the $\beta$ 1,4 linked glucose polymer, cellulose, which remains in the intestinal lumen as nondigestible fiber. Pancreatic amylase hydrolyzes starch highly efficiently within the duodenal lumen by attacking the interior $\alpha$ 1,4 links to yield the final oligosaccharide products before a starch meal reaches the jejunum (Figure 1). As an

43

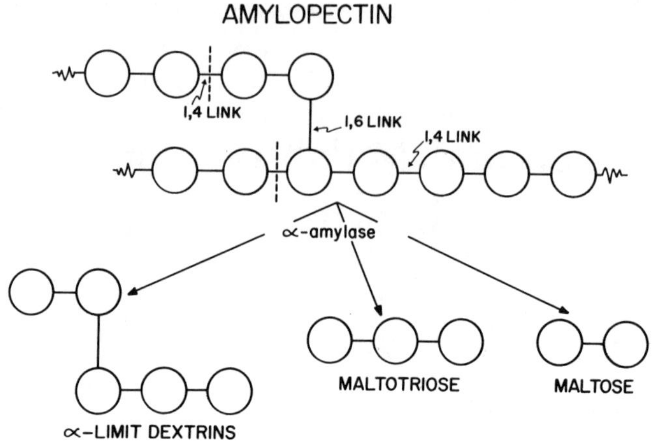

AMYLOPECTIN

**Figure 1.** Action of pancreatic and salivary $\alpha$-amylase on branched starch (amylopectin). A portion of the amylopectin molecule near an $\alpha$ 1,6 branch point is shown. Circles represent glucose units and horizontal links the $\alpha$ 1,4 (maltosyl) linkages; vertical links denote $\alpha$ 1,6 linkage. Since the $\alpha$ 1,6 link and adjacent $\alpha$ 1,4 links are resistant to $\alpha$-amylase action, the $\alpha$-limit dextrins containing 5–8 glucose units are also formed as final products. [From G. M. Gray (1) with permission.]

endoenzyme, amylase cleaves the interior 1,4 links but has very low specificity for the outermost links of the molecule (1). Furthermore, it does not break the 1,6 branching links. For these reasons, the final hydrolytic products of $\alpha$-amylase action are a $(1\rightarrow4)$ linked trisaccharide and a disaccharide having only exterior links (maltotriose and maltose) and the group of branched oligosaccharides containing both $\alpha$ 1,6 and $\alpha$ 1,4 linkages, that is, the $\alpha$-limit dextrins (Figure 1). The formation of oligosaccharide from starch occurs extremely efficiently and is not a rate limiting process in the overall assimilation of starch. The $\alpha$ $(1\rightarrow4)$, $\alpha$ $(1\rightarrow6)$ linked oligosaccharides must be further hydrolyzed by intestinal surface enzymes as detailed below.

## INTESTINAL SURFACE DIGESTION OF OLIGOSACCHARIDES

The final glucosyl oligosaccharide products of intraluminal starch digestion and the disaccharides sucrose and lactose are not assimilated as such across the intestinal mucosal barrier but must first be hydrolyzed on the exterior surface membrane to the constituent monosaccharides. The oligosaccharides of the brush border are integral membrane glycoproteins positioned so that the active hydrolytic site of the molecule is exterior (luminal) to the lipid bilayer of the membrane. As such they act

**Table 1 Intestinal Surface Digestion of Dietary Carbohydrates**

| Carbohydrate Presented | Enzyme | Mechanism of Action | Products |
|---|---|---|---|
| Lactose | Lactase | Hydrolysis of $\beta$ 1,4 linkage of disaccharide (but not of cellulose) | Glucose, galactose |
| Sucrose | Sucrase[a] | Hydrolysis of $\alpha$ 1,4 linkage | Glucose, fructose |
| Maltose, maltotriose | Glucoamylase | Sequential removal of glucosyl residue from nonreducing end | Glucose |
| $\alpha$-Dextrins (see Fig. 2) | Glucoamylase | Initial removal of $\alpha$ (1→4) linked glucose residues from nonreducing end $--\!\!\to$ | Oligosacchride with terminal $\alpha$ (1→6) linked glucose residue; glucose $--\!\!\to$ |
| | $\alpha$-Dextrinase[b] $--\!\!\to$ | Cleavage of $\alpha$ (1→6) linked glucose stub $--\!\!\to$ | Malto-oligosaccharides; glucose $--\!\!\to$ |
| | Sucrase[a] | Hydrolysis of released malto-oligosaccharides | Glucose |

[a] Sucrase, having $\alpha$ 1,4 glucosidase activity, serves as a very active maltase.

[b] Commonly called "isomaltase"; essential for removal of the $\alpha$ (1→6) linked glucose stub from partially hydrolyzed $\alpha$-dextrins.

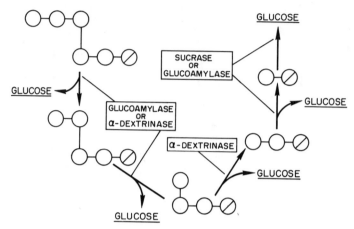

**Figure 2.** Mechanism of sequential removal of glucosyl reidues from an $\alpha$-limit dextrin by complimentary action of membrane oligosaccharidases. Symbols are the same as in Figure 1 and o indicates reducing glucose unit. [Based on G. M. Gray and co-workers (2).]

on their oligosaccharide substrates when contact is made at the luminal surface. The disaccharides are cleaved to their constituent monosaccharide products (Table 1). Larger oligosaccharide products of luminal starch digestion are hydrolyzed in a specific manner by sequential removal of a glucose unit from one end of the molecule. Thus, maltotriose is broken down to maltose and then to glucose and the $\alpha$-dextrins are cleaved by complementary action of three different enzymes acting at discrete regions of the saccharide (2). As outlined in Figure 2, an $\alpha$-dextrin hexasaccharide is converted in sequence to the pentasaccharide and tetrasaccharide by action of either glucoamylase or $\alpha$-dextrinase (commonly called isomaltase). The $\alpha$ 1,6 linked glucose stub can then be removed only by $\alpha$-dextrinase, and the final maltotriose and maltose appear to be attacked by glucoamylase or sucrase, both of which serve as potent maltases.

This surface hydrolysis of oligosaccharides occurs very efficiently so that a slight excess of monosaccharide is released for transport across the intestinal cell. The final monosaccharide transport becomes the rate limiting step in the overall assimilation of most carbohydrates. There is one exception to this, however; lactose is broken down more slowly than other oligosaccharides and, consequently, insufficient glucose and galactose are released for subsequent monosaccharide uptake (3). Hence, the hydrolysis of lactose becomes rate limiting for the overall assimilation of lactose. Despite the relatively rapid nature of surface hydrolysis at the

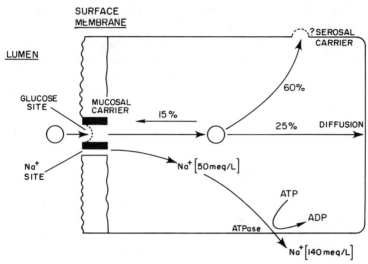

**Figure 3.** Diagram of the mechanisms facilitating the uphill movement of glucose from the intestinal lumen across the intestinal cell to the intercellular spaces. The symbol O denotes free glucose molecule. Based on original Crane hypothesis (4) and recent work of Kimmich (5).

lumen–cell interface for most carbohydrates, large amounts of monosaccharides do not accumulate in the intestinal lumen. This suggests that there may be some regulation of surface digestion, depending upon the ability of the transport mechanism to take up the final monosaccharide products. Indeed, released monosaccharides do cause an inhibition of the intestinal oligosaccharidases and of oligosaccharide hydrolysis in vivo (4). In this way excess quantities of monosaccharide products that might produce an osmotic diarrhea are not allowed to build up in the intestinal contents.

The intestinal membrane oligosaccharidases can be classified as α-glucosidases (sucrase (5), glucoamylase (6), and α-dextrinase (2), see Table 1) and a β-galactosidase (lactase) (7). All are large glycoproteins of greater than 200,000 daltons. Although they are undoubtedly synthesized within the intestinal cell and subsequently inserted into the surface membrane, the details of the process have not been defined. The regulation of oligosaccharidases is a dynamic process since their half-life is only 4 to 16 hours and therefore maintenance of activity at the intestinal surface requires several cycles of synthesis and degradation during the 3 or 4 day life of the human intestinal cell. Sucrase activity is known to increase appreciably with sucrose feeding (8) or in diabetes mellitus (9), probably because the substrate somehow protects the enzyme from the usual degradative process. Degradation of these membrane enzymes probably occurs by action of luminal pancreatic proteases to cleave the enzyme at its anchoring point at the surface of the membrane (10). The overlying surface coat (glycocalyx) may provide some protection against protease action to prevent immediate and wanton destruction at all levels of the intestinal villus, but its role in maintenance of the oligosaccharidases has not been defined.

## TRANSPORT OF FINAL MONOSACCHARIDES

The principal final product released by surface digestion of dietary carbohydrate is glucose. Lesser amounts of galactose (from lactose hydrolysis) and fructose (from sucrose) are also formed. These monosaccharides would not be capable of traversing the hydrophobic brush border membrane except for the presence of specific transport processes. Fructose appears to utilize an entry mechanism that allows its uptake from high luminal to low intracellular concentrations, that is, so-called facilitated diffusion.

Glucose and galactose, having a nearly identical structure, utilize a specific uphill transport process, as shown schematically in Figure 3. This mechanism allows rapid intestinal assimilation of monosaccharide to yield intracellular concentrations appreciably higher than those in the intestinal lumen. Kinetic studies indicate that the uphill component occurs by virtue of a brush border "carrier," probably an integral membrane protein, which has a high affinity for both glucose and sodium ion (Na+) (11, 12). This concept is supported by the recent finding that artificial lipid membrane vesicles containing brush border membrane proteins are capable of pumping glucose into their interior space (13). The mechanism of movement across the brush border membrane is not defined, but it is likely, based on a one-to-one stoichiometric relationship of glucose and Na+ uptake, that both moieties move through hydrophilic channels within the membrane carrier protein (Figure 3). After glucose and Na+ move to the interior surface of the membrane, their affinity for the carrier apparently decreases markedly and they are released within the cytosol. The driving force for the uphill movement of glucose actually occurs indirectly by virtue of the sodium pump at the basolateral membrane, which actively extrudes Na+ into the intercellular space. Based on recent studies with isolated intestinal cells (12), glucose appears to exit from the cell by three separate routes (Figure 3). A small

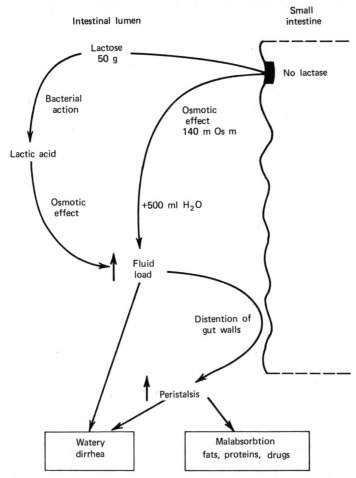

**Figure 4.** Mechanism of carbohydrate intolerance produced by failure of a dietary oligosaccharide to be hydrolyzed on the intestinal surface membrane.

proportion (15%) is extruded back into the lumen by reverse transport via the brush border carrier. The bulk of the glucose appears to exit by a sodium-independent carrier system located at the basolateral membrane; a smaller amount (25%) diffuses passively from the basolateral regions of the cell. Despite its importance for glucose transport, the $Na^+$ pump per se may not be sufficient to explain the rapid uphill movement of monosaccharide. It is likely that membrane electric potentials that develop may provide an additional driving force for intestinal glucose-galactose transport. Whatever the exact combination of processes re-

Table 2    Prevalence of Lactase Deficiency in Healthy Populations[a, b]

| Group | Lactase Deficient (%) |
|---|---|
| North American (white) | 5–20 |
| North American (black) | 70–75 |
| African Bantu | 50 |
| Puerto Rican | 21 |
| Danish | 3 |
| Asians | |
| Filipino | 95 |
| Indian | 55 |
| Thai | 97 |
| Chinese | 87 |
| Eskimo (Greenland) | 88 |
| Nigerian | |
| Yoruba | 99 |
| Fulani | 58 |
| Israeli Jews[c] | 61 |
| Israeli Arabs | 81 |
| Mexican | 74 |

[a] Data from (14).
[b] Lactase activity below 1.0 U/g tissue or 15 U/g protein or blood glucose rise less than 20 mg/100 ml after ingestion of 50 g lactose accompanied by abdominal symptoms and diarrhea. In some instances, percentages given may differ from those in the reference.
[c] Includes Ashkenzi, Sephardi, Iraquis, Yemenite, and Oriental groups with deficiency rates of 44–84%.

sponsible for monosaccharide absorption, uptake is efficient and complete so that no significant dietary carbohydrate escapes being assimilated by the time it reaches the lower jejunum.

## MALDIGESTION AND MALABSORPTION OF CARBOHYDRATE

As outlined above, the assimilation of dietary carbohydrates occurs in a sequential manner beginning with intraluminal digestion (of starch), followed by hydrolysis of oligomers at the intestinal surface membrane, and culminating in transport across the intestine of the final monosaccharide products. A defect at any stage of assimilation can produce an osmotic diarrhea due to retention of the unabsorbed carbohydrates in the intestinal lumen. A schematic diagram of the pathogenesis of carbohydrate malabsorption and intolerance is shown in Figure 4. The carbo-

**Table 3    Secondary Disaccharidase Deficiency in Diseases**[a]

| Condition | Lactase Deficient (%) | Sucrase Deficient (%) | Maltase Deficient (%) |
|---|---|---|---|
| Celiac sprue | | | |
| Mild | 25 | 0 | 0 |
| Moderate | 100 | 80 | 20 |
| Severe | 100 | 100 | 75 |
| Kwashiorkor | 80 | 50 | 30 |
| Tropical sprue | 100 | 65 | 68 |
| Cholera | | | |
| Acute | 86 | 57 | 20 |
| Convalescent | 86 | 0 | 0 |

[a] Modified from G. M. Gray, In P. L. Altman and D. D. Katz, Eds., *Human Health and Disease*, FASEB, Bethesda, Maryland, pp. 124–125.

hydrate attracts water by osmosis to maintain an intraluminal osmolality equal to that in extracellular fluids, and the offending carbohydrate is eventually metabolized by bacteria in lower ileum and colon to smaller fragments that further increase the osmotic effect, and also to hydrogen and carbon dioxide gases. Not surprisingly, patients complain of fullness, rumbling sounds, and abdominal distention followed by increased flatus production and watery diarrhea a few minutes to several hours after ingestion of carbohydrate. Children often become nauseated and may vomit.

## Intestinal Oligosaccharidase Deficiency

Oligosaccharidase deficiency, usually called disaccharidase deficiency, is the most common cause of carbohydrate malabsorption worldwide. Generalized oligosaccharidase deficiency secondary to intestinal disease and the hypolactasia that develops in most of the world's population groups are commonly encountered in clinical practice in the United States. With the exception of the North American white, northern European, and Scandinavian groups, most people develop low lactose levels between 3 years of age and puberty (14). Table 2 lists many of the world's population groups and the prevalence of lactase deficiency among them. The development of lactose intolerance is often anticipated in population groups prone to hypolactasia, and milk ingestion is usually curtailed. Lactase deficiency is more likely to be unrecognized when it occurs acutely as a result of intestinal injury. Patients may experience an acute intestinal illness followed in convalescence by watery diarrhea, which can be shown to abate when milk products are eliminated.

As might be expected, secondary disaccharidase deficiency often occurs in association with other established diseases of the gastrointestinal tract (Table 3). Lactase deficiency secondary to intestinal illness may persist long after the primary disease itself apparently has been cured.

A recessively inherited defect, sucrase deficiency, may not be as rare as originally believed, since it has been relatively easy to identify several families with complaints typical of those found in the irritable colon syndrome which are found to be caused by sucrose intolerance. Radioimmunoassay of intestinal mucosa from patients with sucrase deficiency has shown total absence of the sucrase protein (15), suggesting that there is a regulatory genetic defect that interferes with translation of the sucrase protein before it can acquire its normal three-dimensional configuration. The absence of an inactive enzyme variant probably precludes attempts at inducing the enzyme by dietary means in these patients.

The diagnosis of intestinal oligosaccharidase deficiency can be made definitively by enzymatic assay of as little as 1 mg of a small intestinal biopsy. Since the average diagnostic biopsy obtained for histolopathy is 10–25 mg, it is not necessary to remove additional tissue for the assay. Nevertheless, many patients with chronic diarrhea do not require a peroral intestinal biopsy and two new noninvasive techniques appear to be very useful in establishing the diagnosis of oligosaccharidase deficiency. Both of these tests involve determination of expired metabolic products in the breath. The $^{14}$C-sugar test requires ingestion of only 5 $\mu$C of radioactivity followed by nonquantitative collection of breath over 4 hours (16). Patients with deficiency of the related oligosaccharidase excrete much less $^{14}$CO$_2$ than normal individuals because of the markedly reduced assimilation and subsequent metabolism of the test sugar. The hydrogen breath test is based on the fact that colonic bacteria produce the gas from unabsorbed saccharide remaining in the intestinal lumen. The excess hydrogen is absorbed and excreted in the breath, where it can be collected and analyzed by gas liquid chromatography. Hydrogen excretion rates are typically 2–8 times normal after ingestion of the offending saccharide (17). This test has the added advantage of not exposing the patient to a radioisotope and it is now being used extensively in clinical evaluation of carbohydrate malabsorption.

## REFERENCES

1. G. M. Gray, Carbohydrate digestion and absorption, *New Engl. J. Med.*, **292**, 1225 (1975).
2. G. M. Gray, B. C. Lally, and K. A. Conklin, Action of intestinal sucrase-isomaltase and its free monomers on $\alpha$-limit dextrin, *J. Biol. Chem.*, **254**, 6038 (1979).

3. G. M. Gray and N. A. Santiago, Disaccharide absorption in normal and diseased human intestine, *Gastroenterology*, **51**, 489 (1966).

4. D. H. Alpers and M. N. Cote, Inhibition of lactose hydrolysis by dietary sugars, *Am. J. Physiol.*, **221**, 865 (1971).

5. K. A. Conklin, K. M. Yamashiro, and G. M. Gray, Human intestinal sucrase-isomaltase. Identification of free sucrase and isomaltase and cleavage of the hybird into active distinct subunits, *J. Biol. Chem.*, **250**, 5735 (1975).

6. J. J. Kelly and D. H. Alpers, Properties of human intestinal glucoamylase, *Biochim. Biophys. Acta*, **315**, 113 (1973).

7. G. M. Gray and N. A. Santiago, Intestinal β-galactosidases. I. Separation and characterization of three enzymes in normal human intestine, *J. Cin. Invest.* **48**, 716 (1969).

8. N. S. Rosensweig and R. H. Herman, Control of jejunal sucrase and maltase activity by dietary sucrose of fructose in man: a model for the study of enzyme regulation in man, *J. Clin. Invest.*, **47**, 2253 (1968).

9. W. A. Olsen and H. Korsmo, The intestinal brush border membrane in diabetes, *J. Clin. Invest.*, **60**, 181 (1977).

10. D. H. Alpers and F. J. Tedesco, The possible role of pancreatic proteases in the turnover of intestinal brush border proteins, *Biochim. Biophys. Acta*, **401**, 28 (1975).

11. R. K. Crane, Na+-dependent transport in the intestine and other animal tissue, *Fed. Proc.*, **24**, 1000 (1965).

12. G. A. Kimmich and C. Carter-Su, Membrane potentials and the energetics of intestinal Na+ dependent transport systems, *Am. J. Physiol.*, **235**, C78 (1978).

13. R. K. Crane, P. Malathi, and H. Preiser, Reconstitution of specific sodium-dependent D-glucose transport in liposomes by Triton X-100 extracted proteins from purified brush border membranes, *Biochem. Biophys. Res. Comm.*, **71**, 1010 (1976).

14. G. M. Gray, Intestinal Disaccharidase Deficiencies and Glucose-Galactose Malabsorption, in J. B. Stabury, J. B. Wyngaarden, and D. S. Frederickson, Eds., *Metabolic Basis of Inherited Disease*, 4th ed., McGraw-Hill, New York, 1978, pp. 1526–1536.

15. G. M. Gray, K. A. Conklin, and R. R. W. Townley, Sucrase-isomaltase deficiency. Absence of an inactive enzyme variant, *New Engl. J. Med.*, **294**, 750 (1976).

16. Y. Sasaki, M. Ito, H. Kameda, H. Ueda, T. Aoyagi, N. L. Christopher, T. M. Bayless, and N. H. Wagner, Measurement of [14]C-lactose absorption in the diagnosis of lactase deficiency, *J. Lab. Clin. Med.*, **76**, 824 (1970).

17. A. D. Newcomer, D. B. McGill, P. J. Thomas, and A. F. Hoffman, Prospective comparison of indirect methods for detecting lactase deficiency, *New Engl. J. Med.*, **293**, 1232 (1975).

# 4

# Role of Small Intestine in Digestion of Protein to Amino Acids and Peptides for Transport to Portal Circulation

SIAMAK A. ADIBI, M.D., PH.D.

The University of Pittsburgh School of Medicine, Pittsburgh, Pennsylvania

Man, like any other animal species, depends on a large-scale dietary supply of amino acids for growth, development, multiplication, and metabolic functions. Proteins are essentially the source of amino acids in nature. The breakdown of proteins to constituent amino acids is necessary before we can derive any nutritional or metabolic benefit from their consumption in our daily diet. An important and critical function of the gastrointestinal tract is the delivery of amino acid constituents of these proteins, as free amino acids, to the portal circulation.

During the past two decades, studies in several laboratories have brought new light to our understanding of this function. The purpose of this chapter is to highlight the new concepts, with their supportive evidence, pertaining to digestion and absorption of dietary proteins in human intestine. The breakdown of dietary proteins to free amino acids is achieved in three phases, with the initial phase in the gut lumen, the intermediate phase on the surface membrane of the mucosal epithelium, and the final phase within the mucosal cytoplasm.

The studies of the author described in this review article were supported by a grant from the National Institute of Arthritis, Metabolism, and Digestive Diseases (AM-15861).

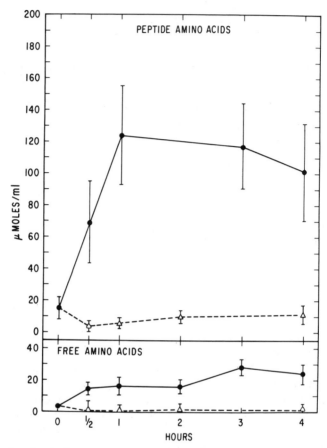

**Figure 1.** Intraluminal concentration (mean ± S.E.M.) of amino acids in peptide (upper panel) and free form (lower panel) before and after a protein-rich (solid line) and a protein-free (dotted line) meal in the jejunum of four human subjects (1).

## INTRALUMINAL PHASE

The main event in the intraluminal phase is the digestion of proteins by pancreatic proteolytic enzymes. The gastric proteolytic enzymes appear to play a minor role in this regard. The products of this digestion are amino acids, and oligopeptides, mostly dipeptides, tripeptides, and tetrapeptides (1). The hydrolytic activity of intraluminal fluid against these oligopeptides is weakly detectable, at best, and is certainly not sufficient to account for their digestion in the lumen (2–6).

Until recently, two dogmas prevailed in the concept of protein digestion. First, digestion is very rapid and almost complete by the time meal proteins reach the upper jejunum (7, 8). Second, there is a large amount of endogenous protein in the gut, which overwhelms the amino acid contribution of dietary proteins to the pool of amino acids in the gut lumen (9).

Evidence controverting the first dogma was provided by our studies which determined directly the fate of a protein (bovine serum albumin) in the gut lumen. When we fed 50 g of this protein in a well-balanced meal to healthy human volunteers, we found that protein digestion was still incomplete as late as 4 hours after the meal, and that the ileum was involved in this process (1). Subsequent to our study, Chung and co-workers (10), using the same test meal, confirmed these results and extended our observations by providing quantitative data on the extent of protein digestion in the intestine of healthy human volunteers. They found that 60% of the meal protein was digested in the upper small intestine and the remainder in the distal small intestine, with the whole process taking more than 4 hours to complete. They also concluded that the ileum is important for the completion of protein digestion in man (10).

Evidence against the second dogma was provided when we compared the intraluminal concentrations of amino acids in free and peptide forms in the intestine of human volunteers after ingestion of two test meals, which were identical in all respects except for their protein composition (1). One meal lacked protein, and the other contained 50 g of bovine serum albumin. As shown in Figure 1, when the meal contained protein there were marked increases in jejunal concentrations of amino acids, both in free and in peptide form. In contrast, when the meal lacked protein the jejunal concentrations of amino acids, both in free and in peptide form, were either decreased or remained unchanged (Figure 1). Similar changes were also observed in the ileum (1), but increases in amino acid and peptide concentrations were not as pronounced as those in the jejunum (Figure 1).

An unexpected finding in the above experiments was the observation that after a protein meal there is a more dramatic increase in the concentration of amino acids in peptide than in free form in human intestine. This observation, which has been confirmed and extended by Chung and co-workers (10), was actually the stimulus for the initiation of our studies on intestinal transport of oligopeptides in man over a decade ago.

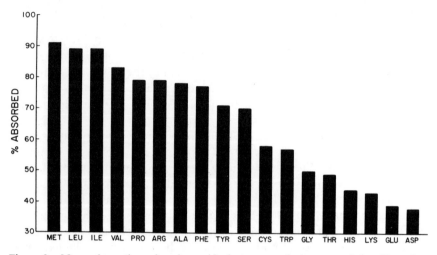

**Figure 2.** Mean absorption of amino acids from test solutions containing 18 amino acids, each at a concentration of 8mM, infused into the jejunum of three human subjects (12).

## SURFACE MEMBRANE PHASE

Although it has been shown that pancreatic enzymes may bind superficially to the brush border membrane of intestinal epithelium, the participation of membrane-bound pancreatic proteolytic enzymes in the process of protein digestion has not yet been established. Whether they participate or not, the fact remains that after a protein meal the brush border membrane is bathed with a mixture of amino acids and oligopeptides. The brush border membrane clears these products of protein digestion by several independent uptake mechanisms and by hydrolysis of the oligopeptides that otherwise cannot be transported intact to absorbable products.

### Amino Acid Transport

The brush border membrane of the small intestine contains at least two distinct active transport systems, one for neutral amino acids and the other for basic amino acids. Although the existence of several different carrier systems for neutral amino acids in human intestine has been suggested, this has not yet been firmly established. This problem has been recently reviewed (11).

When the jejunum of healthy volunteers was perfused with test solutions containing equal concentrations of the 18 common dietary amino

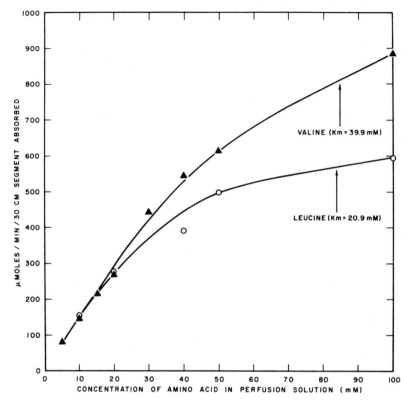

**Figure 3.** Mean absorption rates of leucine and valine from test solutions containing either leucine or valine infused into the jejunum of five to nine human subjects (13).

acids, a highly selective pattern of absorption was obtained (12). The technique of intestinal perfusion and methods of analysis and calculation of absorption rates have been described elsewhere (12, 13). Methionine, leucine, isoleucine, and valine displayed the highest, and glutamic acid and aspartic acid the lowest rates of absorption, with other amino acids being between these two extremes (Figure 2). This pattern of selective absorption appears to be related to differences in the affinity of individual amino acids for carrier systems, interactions between individual amino acids during transport, and presence or absence of electrical charges in the side chain.

The length of side chain is an important factor in determining affinity of neutral amino acids for their carrier system; the longer the side chain the greater the affinity (13). For example, leucine and valine have identical molecular structure except that the side chain of valine is shorter by one carbon atom. As shown in Figure 3, when the jejunum of human volunteers was perfused with a range of concentrations of valine and leucine, saturation of leucine absorption was achieved at a perfusion concentration that was smaller than that for valine. The calculation of $K_m$ (concentration which produces one-half of the maximal absorption rate) by the Lineweaver-Burk analysis of absorption kinetics showed that the $K_m$ of valine is twice that of leucine (39.9 versus 20.9 mM, $p < 0.01$). The apparent $K_m$ value is regarded as an index of affinity for absorption site —the lower the $K_m$ value, the higher the affinity.

The rate of absorption of an amino acid is also influenced by the presence of other amino acids in the gut lumen (14). Amino acids with high affinity for the membrane carrier system inhibit absorption of amino acids with lower affinity (e.g., leucine versus glycine or alanine versus glycine). This inhibition appears to be due to competition for uptake by a carrier system that transports both amino acids (15). In addition to the above type of interaction, there could be stimulation of transport of basic amino acids by the neutral amino acids (16). The mechanism of stimulation apparently is not related to interaction at the level of carrier system in brush border membrane, but is due to interaction within the cell (16). It is well known that charged molecules are less rapidly transported than noncharged molecules across biological membranes. This is consistent with the observations that the basic amino acid carrier system is less efficient than the neutral amino acid carrier system in human intestine (17). These principles may account for the observation that lysine, glutamic acid, and aspartic acid were least absorbed from the amino acid mixture (Figure 2). The relatively high rate of arginine absorption from the amino acid mixture (Figure 2) may reflect a stimulation of transport of this amino acid by a neutral amino acid as discussed above.

## Peptide Transport

For a long time it was believed that complete hydrolysis of proteins to free amino acids in the gut lumen is required for assimilation by intestine. Although in 1953 Agar and co-workers (18) and in 1959 Wiggans and Johnston (19) and Newey and Smyth (20) had unequivocally demonstrated absorption of unhydrolyzed glycylglycine, this observation was not regarded as having very much physiological relevance. It was argued that unlike other dipeptides, glycylglycine is uncommon in dietary proteins, it is exceptionally small, and it is resistant to hydrolysis (21). In 1968, Matthews and co-workers, studying transport in rat intestine (22), and we, studying transport in human intestine (23), independently came to the conclusion that intact absorption is not peculiar to glycylglycine

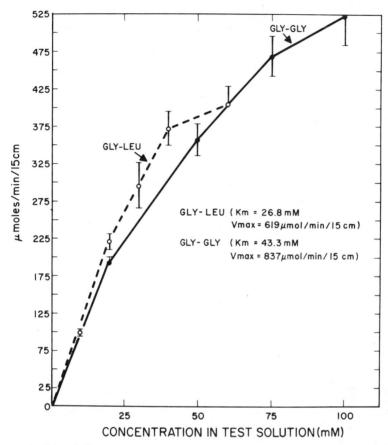

**Figure 4.** Jejunal disappearance rates (mean ± S.E.M.) of glycylglycine and gylcyl-leucine as a function of test solution concentration in five human subjects (24).

but includes other dipeptides. Soon after, several groups of investigators demonstrated intact absorption for a wide variety of dipeptides in both animal and human intestine (21). By early 1970 the question was no longer whether there is absorption of dipeptides, but whether it is physiologically an important mode of dipeptide assimilation in the intestine. In other words, quantitatively, how much of a dipeptide load disappears by intact absorption when introduced into the gut lumen and how much of it disappears by amino acid absorption following brush border peptide hydrolysis? To answer this question, we performed a series of studies using glycylglycine and glycyl-L-leucine as model dipeptides. The goals of these studies were to investigate: (a) kinetics of intestinal disappear-

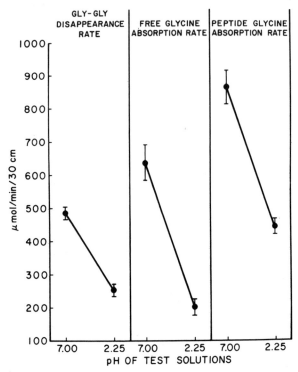

**Figure 5.** Rates of glycylglycine disappearance from test solutions containing 40 mM dipeptide (left panel), rates of glycine absorption from test solutions containing 80 mM free glycine (middle panel), and rates of glycine absorption from solutions containing 40 mM glycylglycine (right panel). Solutions initially had a pH of 7.00. After studies of disappearance and absorption rates were completed, the pH was changed to 2.25, and studies of the disappearance and absorption rates were repeated. The perfusion studies were performed in the jejunum of six human subjects (25).

ance of two dipeptides that differ greatly in their rates of hydrolysis by mucosal peptidases, (b) rates of absorption of the glycine residues of glycylglycine and glycylleucine when the absorption of free glycine is inhibited, (c) rates of dipeptide disappearance when the activity of brush border peptide hydrolases is inhibited, and (d) rates of dipeptide disappearance when dipeptide absorption is inhibited.

*Kinetics of dipeptide disappearance.* When examined in vitro the rate of hydrolysis of glycylleucine by brush border peptide hydrolases is much greater than that of glycylglycine. However, as shown in Figure 4, there was no significant difference in vivo between the rates of glycylglycine and glycylleucine disappearance over the range of perfusion concentra-

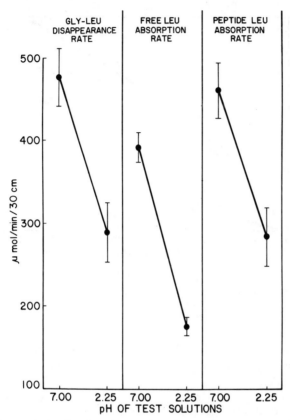

**Figure 6.** Rates of glycylleucine disappearance from test solutions containing 40 mM dipeptide (left panel), rates of leucine absorption from test solutions containing 40 mM free leucine (middle panel), and rates of leucine absorption from test solutions containing 40 mM glycylleucine (right panel). Solutions initially had a pH of 7.00. After the studies of the disappearance and absorption rates were completed, the pH was changed to 2.25, and the studies of the disappearance and absorption rates were repeated. These perfusion studies were performed in the jejunum of six human subjects (25).

tion of 10–60 mM. In fact, the rate of glycylleucine disappearance reached a plateau around the infusion concentration of 40 mM but that of glycylglycine continued to increase at higher infusion concentrations. Kinetic analysis by Lineweaver-Burk plots showed (24) that the maximal rate ($V_{max}$) of glycylglycine absorption was significantly greater than that of glycylleucine (837 ± 62 versus 619 ± 85 $\mu$moles/minute/15 cm segment, $p < 0.01$). These data show that the rates of luminal disappearance of

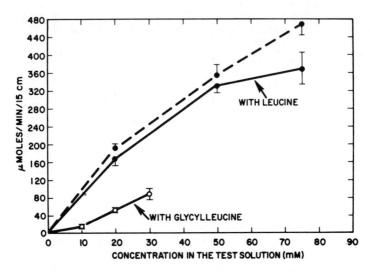

**Figure 7.** Jejunal absorption rates (mean ± S.E.M.) of glycylglycine with or without addition of free leucine (100 mM) or glycylleucine (50 mM) to the test solutions. The broken line represents the absorption curve for glycylglycine without the addition of either free leucine or glycylleucine (24).

these dipeptides do not reflect the characteristics of the hydrolytic system and, therefore, by inference must reflect characteristics of the absorptive system.

*Effect of inhibition of glycine absorption.* As discussed above, leucine and isoleucine inhibit absorption of glycine. We took advantage of this fact to determine whether glycine uptake from glycylglycine or glycylleucine would be remarkably reduced when the amino acid carrier system was saturated with leucine or isoleucine. In other words, if there is hydrolysis of appreciable amounts of these dipeptides by the membrane-bound peptide hydrolases, the addition of leucine to a glycylglycine solution or the addition of isoleucine to a glycylleucine solution should result in a profound inhibition of glycine absorption from these dipeptide solutions. The results of these experiments showed that jejunal absorption of the glycine residues of the above dipeptides was minimally or not at all reduced when the amino acid carrier system was saturated by either leucine or isoleucine (2).

*Effect of inhibition of peptide hydrolase.* Several studies have clearly established that acidification impairs the activity of peptide hydrolases (25). In fact, there is very little, if any, hydrolysis when the pH is lower than 6. Taking advantage of this fact, we investigated the jejunal disappearance rates of glycylglycine and glycylleucine when the pH of per-

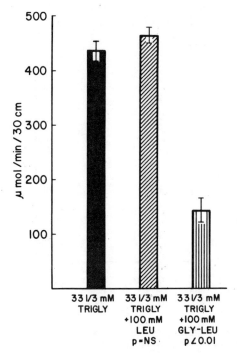

**Figure 8.** Disappearance rates of triglycine when test solutions contained only tri-glycine ($33\frac{1}{3}$ mM), or triglycine together with 100 mM leucine, or triglycine together with 100 mM glycylleucine. These perfusion studies were performed in the jejunum of four human subjects (3).

fusion solutions was either 7.00 or 2.25 (25). When solutions of pH 7.00 were used, the intraluminal pH was maintained near neutrality, but when solutions of pH 2.25 were used, the intraluminal pH became markedly acidic (around 3.0). Despite such high acidity in the gut lumen, there was still considerable absorption of both glycylglycine and glycyl-leucine (Figures 5 and 6). The magnitude of reduction in absorption at acidic pH was only 38% for glycylleucine and 48% for glycylglycine. These reductions did not appear to be related to impaired hydrolysis, since under the same experimental conditions (Figures 5 and 6) the ab-sorptions of glycine and leucine, which are not dependent on hydrolysis, showed greater reductions (55–68%). Dipeptides and amino acids have free carboxyl and amino groups and, therefore, are subject to protona-tion effects. When the environmental pH is changed from neutral to acidic, amino acids and dipeptides will be converted to a monovalent cationic form. The above mode of molecular alteration appeared to be

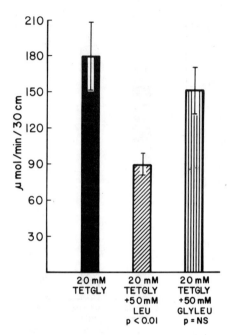

**Figure 9.** Disappearance rates of tetraglycine when test solutions contained only tetraglycine (20 mM), tetraglycine together with 50 mM leucine, or tetraglycine together with 50 mM glycylleucine. These perfusion studies were performed in the jejunum of four human subjects (4).

the principal reason for the reduction in the absorption of free amino acids and dipeptides. This impression was supported by the observation that the reduction in absorption is less severe for amino acid constituents of dipeptides than for the same amino acids in free form. Apparently, the peptide bond protects the amino group of the amino acid residue in the C-terminal position from the protonation effect.

That inhibition of peptide hydrolase activity does not significantly alter the dipeptide disappearance rate was also supported by another observation. Entirely by chance during the course of our studies of peptide transport, we found that leucine inhibits the activity of brush border peptide hydrolases (4). This observation has been recently confirmed and extended to the intestinal brush border membrane oligopeptidase of rats (26). As shown in Figure 7, leucine in high concentrations had no significant effect on luminal disappearance rates of glycylglycine.

*Effect of inhibition of peptide absorption.* Intestinal brush border membrane has very little hydrolytic activity against glycylglycine, and, furthermore, this activity is not very much affected by the addition of glycylleucine to an enzyme reaction mixture. However, the jejunal disappearance rate of glycylglycine was markedly (70–80%) inhibited when glycylleucine was added to the perfusion solution. The kinetic analysis of this inhibition by Lineweaver-Burk plot revealed that inhibition was competitive in nature (24).

In summary, considering all of the above data compels one to conclude that intact absorption is the major mode and hydrolysis the minor mode of disappearance of these dipeptides in human jejunum. Furthermore, the data suggest that a carrier system is involved in the absorption of dipeptides. Indeed, we have already characterized the function of this carrier system in human jejunum (24). The essential features of this carrier system are as follows:

1. It does not take up amino acids, but transports dipeptides.
2. It has a higher maximal rate of uptake than the amino acid carrier system.
3. It prefers dipeptides with lipophilic amino acids in both the N- and the C-terminal position.

The demonstration of dipeptide absorption prompted us to question whether tripeptides are also assimilated in this manner in human intestine. To investigate this possibility, we studied the mechanism of luminal disappearance rates of two tripeptides, namely triglycine and trileucine (3). Among the 8000 theoretically possible tripeptides containing the 20 possible amino acids found in protein, these two tripeptides represent the spectrum of water solubility and molecular size. Triglycine is much more water soluble and much smaller than triluecine.

As shown in Figure 8, leucine, the inhibitor of brush border peptide hydrolases, had no significant effect on the disappearance rate of triglycine in the jejunum. In contrast, when glycylleucine, an inhibitor of dipeptide absorption, was added to the triglycine solution, the luminal disappearance of this tripeptide was markedly reduced (Figure 8). These data indicate that luminal disappearance of triglycine is principally by intact absorption and, furthermore, this absorption is mediated by the same carrier system that transports dipeptides. Similar studies with trileucine showed that luminal disappearance of this tripeptide occurs mostly by hydrolysis to leucine and dileucine (3). Leucine and dileucine are then transported by amino acid and peptide transport systems, respectively.

After tripeptides, the question arises regarding the intestinal fate of tetrapeptides. We reasoned that among the 160,000 theoretically possible tetrapeptides, tetraglycine would be the most likely candidate for intact

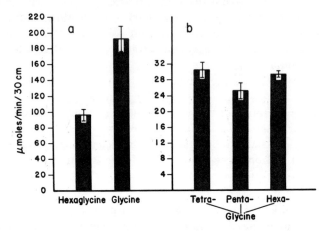

**Figure 10.** (*a*) Rates of glycine absorption from test solutions containing either 3 mM hexaglycine or the equivalent amount of glycine in free form, i.e., 18 mM glycine. The difference is statistically signficant (*p* < 0.01). (*b*) Rates of peptide disappearance from solutions of 3 mM tetraglycine, 3 mM pentaglycine, or 3 mM hexaglycine. All of these perfusion studies were performed in the jejunum of five human subjects (4).

absorption (4). As already discussed, diglycine and triglycine are absorbed intact, and tetraglycine has the smallest molecular size among the tetrapeptides. As shown in Figure 9, leucine markedly inhibited the jejunal disappearance rate of tetraglycine, while glycylleucine had no significant effect on this rate. These data indicate that tetraglycine is not a substrate for the peptide carrier system, and its luminal disappearance is mostly by hydrolysis by the brush border peptide hydrolases. In view of this finding, we considered it unlikely that there would be large-scale intact absorption of other tetrapeptides in human intestine.

## Peptide Hydrolysis

From the above discussion, it becomes evident that oligopeptides with four to six amino acid residues must be hydrolyzed if the assimilation of dietary protein is to be complete. These oligopeptides are resistant to the hydrolytic action of pancreatic enzymes, and there is very little peptide hydrolase activity against them in the gut lumen. Therefore, brush border peptide hydrolases, which have been shown to have efficient hydrolytic capacity against tetrapeptides, pentapeptides, and hexapeptides (27, 28), play a critical role in converting these peptides to absorbable products. Studies from two independent laboratories (29, 30) have resulted in isolation and characterization of up to four peptide hydrolases from the brush border of rat intestine. These enzymes are aminooligopeptidases. In other words, they sequentially release amino acids from the amino terminal position.

Using glycine homologous peptides as model substrates, we investigated (a) whether increases in the number of amino acid residues would affect the rate of hydrolysis of oligopeptides by the brush border enzymes, and (b) whether peptide hydrolysis or transport is a more limiting step. As shown in Figure 10b, under identical experimental conditions, there was no significant difference between the rate of hydrolysis of tetraglycine and pentaglycine or between pentaglycine and hexaglycine. On the other hand, over a wide range of concentrations, rates of luminal disappearance of triglycine (mostly absorption) were always nearly twice the rates of luminal disappearance of tetraglycine (mostly hydrolysis). These data indicate that for glycine peptides, transport is much more efficient than hydrolysis.

### Factors Determining Peptide Transport or Hydrolysis

Intestinal brush border membrane has the capacity for both transport and hydrolysis of many oligopeptides. At least three factors appear to influence which system predominates over the other in luminal disappearance of oligopeptides. First, different affinities of an oligopeptide for binding sites of the peptide transport and the hydrolytic systems may enable the system with the greater affinity to play a greater role in its disappearance from the gut lumen. Second, the $V_{max}$ of brush border peptide hydrolases is achieved at much lower concentrations of substrate than the peptide carrier system. Therefore, it is conceivable that as the luminal concentration of oligopeptides exceeds certain levels, peptide transport may become a more important component of luminal disappearance rates. Third, as discussed above, certain amino acids inhibit the activity of brush border peptide hydrolases. Therefore, such feedback inhibition may limit the potential of the hydrolytic system when the concentration of amino acids in the gut lumen has reached certain critical levels.

### CYTOPLASMIC PHASE

Upon entry into the enterocytes, dipeptides and tripeptides are rapidly hydrolyzed to their constituent amino acids by the cytoplasmic peptide hydrolases. Studies of subcellular distribution of dipeptidase activities have shown that 85–100% of this activity resides in the cytoplasmic region (31–33). With tripeptides as substrates, the peptide hydrolase activity in the brush border becomes more pronounced. In fact, with certain tripeptides, such as trileucine, a substantial percentage of hydrolase activity is associated with the brush border fraction (28). Nevertheless, with other tripeptides, such as triglycine, the peptide hydrolase activity of the cytosol far exceeds that of brush border (28). With tetrapeptides and larger oligopeptides as substrates, the cytoplasmic fraction displays very little activity, and the brush border fraction becomes the principal source of peptide hydrolase activity of the mucosal cells of the small intestine (27, 28, 32). Four peptide hydrolases from the rat intestinal mucosa have been isolated and characterized (34). Although these peptide hydrolases, like those of the brush border region, are amino-oligopeptidases, they are not the same enzymes as those found in the cell membrane. Their biological characteristics, as well as their response to dietary manipulation, are entirely different (31, 35).

With hydrolysis of dipeptides and tripeptides to amino acids within the intestinal mucosal cells, the process of protein digestion reaches completion. Nevertheless, a small fraction of these peptides may escape hydrolysis by the cytoplasmic peptide hydrolases and enter the portal circulation in unhydrolyzed form. Indeed, dipeptides have been shown to appear in portal blood during intestinal perfusion of dipeptides in rats (36). During the perfusion of human intestine with dipeptides, we could not detect glycylleucine in peripheral plasma, but did find a sizable concentration of glycylglycine in peripheral venous blood (2). Much larger tissue dipeptide hydrolase activity (37) and a shorter plasma half-life (38) for glycylleucine than for glycylglycine are probably responsible for the failure to detect the former dipeptide in the peripheral circulation. However, under physiological conditions after a protein meal, probably small amounts of peptides escape hydrolysis by cytoplasmic hydrolases and enter the portal circulation in unhydrolyzed form. Although this problem has not yet been adequately studied in man, there is evidence that after a gelatin meal, hydroxyproline peptides, which are resistant to hydrolysis, may be detected in systemic circulation (39).


## ADVANTAGES OF PEPTIDES OVER AMINO ACIDS FOR ENTERAL NUTRITION

In recent years, there has been increasing use of amino acid formula diets (elemental) for oral feedings in patients with gastrointestinal disorders. For several reasons, dipeptides and tripeptides appear to offer advantages over amino acids for inclusion in such diets:

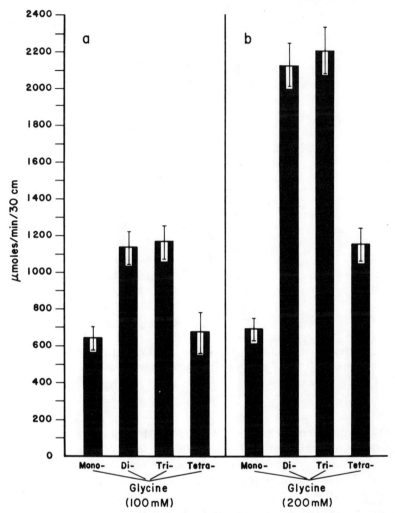

**Figure 11.** Rates of glycine uptake from solutions containing equivalent amounts of glycine in free or peptide form (mean ± S.E.M. in four subjects). (*a*) Rates from 100 mM glycine equivalent solutions; (*b*) rates from 200 mM glycine equivalent solutions (4).

1. Several studies have firmly established that the rates of amino acid absorption from dipeptides and tripeptides and protein hydrolysate solutions are significantly greater than from corresponding solutions of amino acids (2–6, 40–42). To illustrate this phenomenon, the rates of uptake of glycine from glycine, diglycine, triglycine, and tetraglycine solutions are compared in Figure 11. The test solutions contained

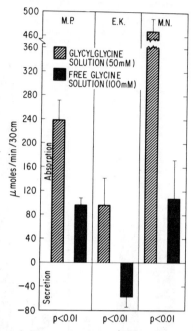

**Figure 12.** Jejunal absorption rates (mean ± S.E.M.) of glycine from test solutions containing equal amounts of glycine in free or dipeptide form in three untreated celiac sprue patients (46).

amounts equivalent to either 100 or 200 mM of glycine. At the glycine equivalent concentration of 100 mM, the rate of glycine uptake from the glycine solution was similar to that from the tetraglycine solution, but it was considerably smaller (nearly half) than the rates of glycine uptake from either diglycine or triglycine solutions. When the concentration of glycine equivalent in the test solution was increased to 200 mM, the rates of glycine uptake from all three peptide solutions were increased, but the rate of glycine uptake from the glycine solution remained unchanged. As a result, the rate of glycine uptake from the diglycine and triglycine solutions was even greater (near fourfold increase) than the rate of uptake from the glycine solution. In another series of studies, we found that this kinetic advantage was no longer apparent when larger peptides, such as hexaglycine, were used. Inasmuch as hexaglycine is not soluble in aqueous solution at concentrations greater than 3 mM, rates of glycine uptake were compared from test solutions containing either 3 mM hexaglycine or 18 mM glycine (Figure 10a). The rate of glycine uptake from the glycine solution was nearly two times that from the hexaglycine solution. The explanations for differences in rates of glycine uptake from solutions of glycine and glycine peptides are detailed elsewhere (4).

2. Elemental diets are usually quite hypertonic. Patients with gastrointestinal disorders usually do not tolerate hypertonic diets. Studies in rats have shown that a single hypertonic force feeding produces jejunal cell loss associated with loss of brush border disaccharidases and focal ultrastructural damage (43). The problem of hypertonicity can be entirely eliminated or considerably reduced by substituting peptides for the amino acid components.

3. Dietary protein and caloric deficiencies and inflammatory diseases of the small intestine cause reduction in jejunal absorption rates of amino acids in human intestine (44–46). In these situations, peptide absorption appears less affected than that of amino acids (47–50). An example of these observations is shown in Figure 12. In three patients with active celiac sprue the jejunal rate of glycine absorption from a 50 mM glycylglycine solution is compared to the rate of glycine absorption from a corresponding glycine solution (100 mM). Normally, there is less than a twofold difference in the rates of glycine uptake from 100 mM glycine and 50 mM glycylglycine infusion solutions (47). In these patients, the difference in rates of glycine uptake from these infusion solutions was increased threefold to sixfold. In fact, in one patient (EK) there was an actual net secretion of glycine into the lumen when the free glycine solution was infused. In contrast, there was glycine absorption when the jejunum of this patient was infused with the glycylglycine test solution.

In summary, the amino acid content of the proteins we consume in our daily diet reaches the portal circulation mostly in the form of free amino acids. There are three phases in the completion of this task. During the initial phase, proteins are hydrolyzed by pancreatic enzymes to amino acids and oligopeptides in the gut lumen. The intermediate phase, which takes place on the brush border membrane of the intestinal mucosa, consists of two components (a) uptake of amino acids, dipeptides, and tripeptides by amino acid and peptide carrier systems, and (b) hydrolysis of oligopeptides to absorbable products. The final phase is the hydrolysis of absorbed dipeptides and tripeptides to amino acids within the mucosal cytoplasm. The fact that the small intestine of man has the capacity for large-scale absorption of dipeptides and tripeptides may have useful clinical application. Patients with digestive and absorptive disorders are usually treated with "elemental diets," which contain free amino acids as a nitrogen source and are generally hypertonic. Substituting dipeptides and tripeptides for the amino acids of these diets may not only improve the absorptive efficiency, but will surely reduce osmotic problems associated with the feeding of elemental diets.

# REFERENCES

1. S. A. Adibi and D. W. Mercer, *J. Clin. Invest.*, **52**, 1586 (1973).
2. S. A. Adibi and E. L. Morse, *J. Clin Invest.*, **50**, 2266 (1971).
3. S. A. Adibi, E. L. Morse, S. S. Masilamani, and P. M. Amin, *J. Clin. Invest.*, **56**, 1355 (1975).
4. S. A. Adibi and E. L. Morse, *J. Clin. Invest.*, **60**, 1008 (1977).
5. D. B. A. Silk, D. Perrett, and M. L. Clark, *Clin. Sci. Molec. Med.*, **45**, 291 (1973).
6. D. B. A. Silk, D. Perrett, J. P. W. Webb, and M. L. Clark, *Clin. Sci. Molec. Med.*, **46**, 393 (1974).
7. B. Borgström, A. Dahlqvist, G. Lundh, and J. Sjövall, *J. Clin. Invest.*, **36**, 1521 (1957).
8. C. W. Crane and A. Neuberger, *Biochem. J.*, **74**, 313 (1960).
9. E. S. Nasset, *Am. J. Diges. Dis.*, **9**, 175 (1964).
10. Y. C. Chung, Y. S. Kim, A. Shadchehr, A. Garrido, I. L. MacGregor, and M. H. Sleisenger, *Gastroenterology*, **72**, A-15 (1977).
11. S. A. Adibi, *Am. J. Clin. Nutr.*, **29**, 205 (1976).
12. S. A. Adibi, S. J. Gray, and E. Menden, *Am. J. Clin. Nutr.*, **20**, 24 (1967).
13. S. A. Adibi, *Gastroenterology*, **56**, 903 (1969).
14. S. A. Adibi and S. J. Gray, *Gastroenterology*, **52**, 837 (1967).
15. B. Fleshler, J. H. Butt, and J. D. Wismar, *J. Clin. Invest.*, **45**, 1433 (1966).
16. J. W. L. Robinson, *European J. Biochem.*, **7**, 78 (1968).
17. M. D. Hellier, B. Chir, C. D. Holdsworth, and D. Perrett, *Gastroenterology*, **65**, 613 (1973).
18. W. T. Agar, F. J. R. Hird, and S. G. Sidhu, *J. Physiol.*, **121**, 255 (1953).
19. D. S. Wiggans and J. M. Johnson, *Biochim. Biophys. Acta*, **32**, 69 (1959).
20. H. Newey and D. H. Smyth, *J. Physiol.*, **145**, 48 (1959).
21. D. M. Matthews, *Physiological Reviews*, **55**, 537 (1975).
22. D. M. Matthews, R. F. Crampton, and M. T. Lis, *Lancet*, **2**, 639 (1968).
23. S. A. Adibi and E. Phillips, *Clin. Res.*, **16**, 446 (1968).
24. S. A. Adibi and M. R. Soleimanpour, *J. Clin. Invest.*, **53**, 1368 (1974).
25. M. R. Fogel and S. A. Adibi, *J. Lab. Clin. Med.*, **84**, 327 (1974).
26. Y. S. Kim and E. J. Brophy, *Gastroenterology*, **76**, 82 (1979).
27. Y. S. Kim, Y. W. Kim, and M. H. Sleisenger, *Biochim. Biophys. Acta*, **370**, 283 (1974).
28. J. A. Nicholson and T. J. Peters, *Clin. Sci. Molec. Med.*, **54**, 205 (1978).
29. F. Wojnarowska and G. M. Gray, *Biochim. Biophys. Acta*, **403**, 147 (1975).
30. C. R. Shoaf, R. M. Berko, and W. D. Heizer, *Biochim. Biophys. Acta*, **445**, 694, (1976).
31. Y. S. Kim, W. Birtwhistle, and Y. W. Kim, *J. Clin. Invest.*, **51**, 1419 (1972).
32. T. J. Peters, *Clin. Sci. Molec. Med.*, **45**, 803 (1973).
33. M. Das and A. N. Radhakrihnan, *Clin. Sci. Molec. Med.*, **46**, 501 (1974).
34. C. M. Schiller, T. Huang, and W. D. Heizer, *Gastroenterology*, **72**, 93 (1977).
35. J. A. Nicholson, D. M. McCarthy, and Y. S. Kim, *J. Clin. Invest.*, **54**, 890 (1974).

36. D. J. Boullin, R. F. Crampton, C. E. Heading, and D. Pelling, *Clin. Sci. Molec. Med.*, 45, 849 (1973).

37. B. A. Krzysik and S. A. Adibi, *Am. J. Physiol.*, 233, E450 (1977).

38. S. A. Adibi, B. A. Krzysik, and A. L. Drash, *Clin. Sci. Molec. Med.*, 52, 193 (1977).

39. D. J. Prockop, H. R. Keiser, and A. Sjoerdsma, *Lancet*, 2, 527 (1962).

40. M. D. Hellier, C. D. Holdsworth, I. McColl, and D. Perrett, *Gut*, 13, 965 (1972).

41. G. C. Cook, *Br. J. Nutr.*, 30, 13 (1973).

42. D. B. A. Silk, T. C. Marrs, J. M. Addison, D. Burston, M. L. Clark, and D. M. Matthews, *Clin. Sci. Molec. Med.*, 45, 715 (1973).

43. S. Teichberg, F. Lifshitz, R. Pergolizzi, and R. A. Wapnir, *Pediat. Res.*, 12, 720 (1978).

44. S. A. Adibi and E. R. Allen, *Gastroenterology*, 59, 404 (1970).

45. H. P. Schedl, C. E. Pierce, A. Rider, J. A. Clifton, and G. Nokes, *J. Clin. Invest.*, 47, 417 (1968).

46. S. A. Adibi, M. R. Fogel, and R. M. Agrawal, *Gastroenterology*, 67, 586 (1974).

47. D. B. A. Silk, P. J. Kumar, D. Perrett, M. L. Clark, and A. M. Dawson, *Gut*, 15, 1 (1974).

48. M. R. Fogel, M. M. Ravitch, and S. A. Adibi, *Gastroenterology*, 71, 729 (1976).

49. M. D. Hellier, A. N. Radhakrishnan, V. Ganapathy, V. I. Mathan, and S. J. Baker, *Gut*, 17, 511 (1976).

50. J. J. Carcino, *Clin. Res.*, 25, 535A (1977).

# 5

# Vitamin D and the Regulation of Calcium Absorption in the Small Intestine

DAVID SCHACHTER, M.D.

Columbia University College of Physicians and Surgeons, New York, New York

One day in May 1960, a house staff officer appeared in my laboratory to begin an elective period of research for 3 months. We had met on the Medical Service of Presbyterian Hospital, where he, the intern, and I, the junior attending, worked closely each day, puzzling over the more complicated clinical cases and trying to guide the medical students. He had impressed me on the clinical service as energetic, scholarly, and articulate, but that first day in the laboratory I did not quite know what to expect: bench-top research is not for everyone. After a short talk in which I outlined some specific research objectives and indicated an experimental method of approach, my new colleague—Dan Kimberg—was off and running. Within hours any apprehensions on my part were gone. It was as though he knew instinctively how to proceed, and day by day I watched the experimental results accumulate. By the end of the 3 month period the observations filled two manuscripts (1, 2) and Dan had launched his extraordinary career in investigation. Not that he did not meet setbacks and problems—he was just determined to overcome them, an essential characteristic of the really great experimenter. One particularly vivid example illustrates this trait. Dan had carefully nurtured three groups of weanling rats on diets containing various levels of calcium, and after 5 weeks he was ready to prepare an everted duodenal gut sac from each animal to test calcium transport in vitro. The preparations went smoothly and the sacs were shaking under oxygen in a large

The research work described here was supported by grant AM-01483 of the National Institute of Arthritis, Metabolic and Digestive Diseases.

Warburg bath when the shaking motor suddenly died and our preparations—so carefully nurtured for 5 weeks—were in imminent danger of anoxia and destruction. Dan grabbed a pair of pliers and mechanically rotated the drive shaft at the prescribed 110 cycles/minute. We took turns acting as human motors for the entire 3 hours of incubation, and the experimental results were among the most clear-cut of our entire study.

There is much more to say about Dan, whose subsequent career touched, enriched, and inspired so many. Other contributors to this volume and others among his students and colleagues will add to the recorded memory of this gifted and giving academic physician. I feel his presence strongly as I write this chapter on the subject that first brought us together and continued to fascinate him throughout his career.

## REGULATION OF BODY CALCIUM

The need to regulate the total store of body calcium becomes evident on considering the disastrous consequences of marked depletion or over-expansion of the stores. Moreover, the body stores must be regulated in the face of the varying requirements of growth and pregnancy, as compared to maintenance, and accomodation must be made to the availability of calcium in the diet. Accordingly, evolution has seen the development of a complex regulatory scheme which we will consider at various levels: the whole organism, organs, cells, and molecules.

The overall balance of calcium involves the interaction of several organ systems as illustrated in Figure 1. A fraction of the daily food calcium is absorbed in the small intestine by a facultative mechanism which varies with the needs of the organism as a whole. The absorption is dependent on vitamin D and the details of this regulatory pathway will be described below. The fraction of food calcium not absorbed in the small intestine appears in the feces along with an additional moiety, the "endogenous fecal calcium," which originates from the endogenous calcium stores. Endogenous fecal calcium gains access to the intestinal lumen via the gastrointestinal secretions and sloughing of intestinal mucosal cells. Unlike the absorption of calcium, the latter processes are not regulated in accord with the body's needs and represent relatively fixed losses that must be balanced each day or the organism goes into negative balance with gradual depletion of body stores. Calcium in the extracellular fluids is in dynamic interchange with the major store of body calcium, the hydroxyapatite of bone. Finally, renal excretion of calcium, which can be modulated in accord with the concentration of the cation in the extra-

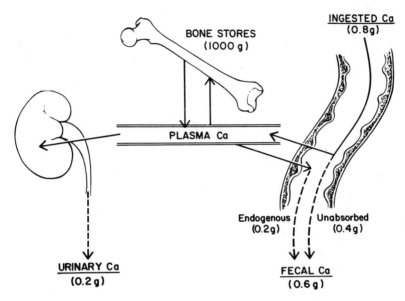

**Figure 1.** Pathways involved in the regulation of calcium balance. Values in parentheses indicate typical quantities of calcium ingested or excreted (g/day) or total bone stores (g) in an adult.

cellular fluid, represents a second major pathway of loss from the body.

For an adult in calcium balance, ingested Ca = excreted Ca = fecal Ca (unabsorbed + endogenous) + urinary Ca + other losses (sweat, etc.). On a daily intake of approximately 800 mg total food Ca, such an adult might absorb approximately one-half and excrete the remainder; endogenous fecal Ca and urinary Ca would then balance the 400 mg absorbed. The quantities listed here are subject to considerable variation, due in part to physiological differences between individuals and in part to different dietary levels of Ca in various geographical regions. As a consequence the recommended dietary allowances for calcium differ somewhat when formulated in the United States (3) as compared to Europe (4).

In this survey we focus on the question of how the small intestine regulates the fraction of dietary calcium absorbed in accord with the needs of the whole body. This regulation was clearly demonstrated in man and experimental animals by the balance studies of Nicolaysen and his collaborators (5). In the decades since these studies were published, we have come to realize that the answer to the question involves the operation of specialized transport mechanisms in the cells that line the lumen of the small intestine, the enterocytes. Moreover, at least four such

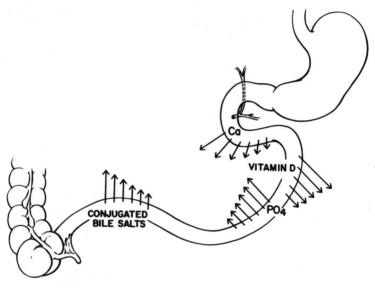

**Figure 2.** Absorptive mechanisms in the small intestine which are essential for maintenance of the bone mineral stores.

specialized mechanisms should be considered from the standpoint of the interrelationship of the small intestine and the bone mineral, an interrelationship that is extremely important in the pathogenesis of osteomalacia related to disease of the digestive tract. Figure 2 shows the mechanisms involved. Calcium is absorbed by an active cation transport mechanism which is dependent on vitamin D. Although this mechanism can be detected in almost all regions of the small intestine, it is maximal in the proximal duodenal mucosa. (In vivo absorption of Ca, on the other hand, may take place mainly in the distal small intestine, where food chyme remains in contact with the mucosa for a longer period.) Maintenance of the calcium pump mechanism requires vitamin D, and the sterol either originates by ultraviolet irradiation of 7-dehydrocholesterol in the skin or is absorbed from food sources in the proximal two-thirds or so of the small intestine. The absorption of the highly apolar vitamin D sterols is by means of the formation of mixed micelles with bile salts in the intestinal lumen. Uptake of the vitamin at the microvillus surface of the enterocyte is followed by the packaging of the sterol with other lipids, including long-chain triglycerides, cholesterol, and cholesterol esters, in chylomicrons, which then pass across the basolateral membranes and into the lymph of the intestinal lacteals. Any interruption of this series of steps leads to lipid malabsorption, depletion of vita-

ENTRY-EXIT MODEL OF CALCIUM TRANSPORT

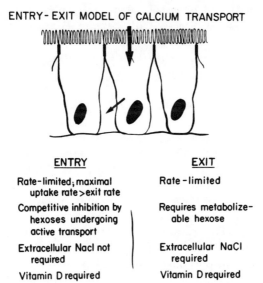

| ENTRY | EXIT |
|---|---|
| Rate-limited; maximal uptake rate >exit rate | Rate-limited |
| Competitive inhibition by hexoses undergoing active transport | Requires metabolize-able hexose |
| Extracellular Nacl not required | Extracellular NaCl required |
| Vitamin D required | Vitamin D required |

**Figure 3.** Entry-exit hypothesis of calcium transport across the enterocyte of the small intestinal mucosa.

min D, and interruption of normal calcium absorption owing to impairment of the cation pump. Gastroenterologists are well aware, for example, that deficits in bile salts lead to calcium malabsorption and osteomalacia. Thus the integrity of the enterohepatic pathway for recirculation of bile salts is essential for normal calcium absorption. As shown in Figure 2, bile salts are normally absorbed via an active anion transport mechanism in the distal ileum (6) and interruption of this process by disease or surgical resection leads to loss of bile salts into the stool. If these losses cannot be matched by increased synthesis of bile salts from cholesterol in the liver, the bile salt concentration in the intestinal lumen may fall below the "critical micellar concentration," lipid and vitamin D absorption are interfered with, and calcium malabsorption results. Finally, studies with rat intestinal preparations in vitro have provided convincing evidence that intestinal absorption of inorganic phosphate, a major component of bone hydroxyapatite, also occurs by means of an active (anion) pump which is maximal in the jejunal mucosa and dependent on vitamin D (7–9).

The result of the operation of the foregoing intestinal transport mechanisms is that extensive disease of any region of the small intestine may result in defective absorption of calcium and phosphate. Ileal disease may compromise bile salt absorption and lead secondarily to malabsorption of vitamin D and hence of calcium and phosphate. Disease of the jejunum can interfere directly with vitamin D and phosphate transfer; Ca absorption is secondarily affected. Duodenal disease may directly involve the region most specialized for Ca transport.

## CELLULAR MECHANISM OF CALCIUM TRANSPORT

The foregoing discussion emphasizes the importance of the intestinal enterocyte in the regulation of calcium absorption and in this section we consider further the nature of the transcellular transport mechanism. Much of our information comes from studies with intestinal preparations in vitro. The results of the work of a number of laboratories have established that Ca transit can occur against electrochemical potential gradients (1, 2, 10–18). This cation pump is relatively specific for calcium as compared to other divalent cations and demonstrates the typical features of other active transport mechanisms: dependence on cell metabolism and oxidative phosphorylation, limitation in the maximal velocity of transport, dependence on the transcellular electrical potential, and competitive inhibition by related substances. More uniquely, the intestinal mechanism has specific features which point to its importance in the regulation of Ca absorption: it is dependent on vitamin D and it varies facultatively with the needs of the organism as modified by growth, pregnancy, and deficiency or excess of calcium in the diet. The molecular mechanisms involved in these regulatory responses are partly known and will be discussed below. Here we describe a cellular model of the calcium transport involving sequential entry and exit steps, that is, transit across the microvillus and basolateral membranes, respectively, of the enterocyte (Figure 3). The model is based on transport experiments with intestinal preparations in vitro (2, 16–18). In these studies entry was defined operationally as net uptake of $Ca^{+2}$ at the mucosal surface and exit as net transport of the cation to the serosal surface of everted duodenal sacs. When estimated at various initial concentrations of calcium, both entry and exit were rate limited, that is, showed saturation kinetics with increasing calcium concentration. However, the maximal rate of entry greatly exceeded that of exit. In addition, the entry step (a) could be inhibited competitively by hexoses undergoing active transport, including glucose, galactose, and 3-methylglucose, (b) did not require NaCl in the mucosal medium, and (c) did require vitamin D. The exit step was identified as an uphill, active transport process and was dependent on the presence of a metabolizable hexose in the medium, such as glucose or fructose, and on extracellular NaCl. Vitamin D was again required for the exit process. Since the maximal velocity of the exit process is less than that of entry, the former appears to be the rate limiting step in the overall transport. Since the development of this hypothesis, considerable information has been obtained on the molecular organization and function of the antipodal microvillus and basolateral membranes. These differ in ultrastructure (19), electrophysiological properties (20), protein components (21), enzyme and transport activities (22, 23), lipid fluidity (24), and lipid composition (24–27). It is hardly surprising that transit of $Ca^{+2}$ across each of these membranes also has different features, and it is noteworthy that regulation may occur at each portal, as suggested by the requirement for vitamin D for each transit step. Finally, it bears emphasis that the model in Figure 3 does not exclude still other discrete transit mechanisms, such as intracellular translocations mediated by organellar membranes. Indeed, evidence has appeared that the Golgi apparatus may be involved in vitamin D-dependent translocation of calcium (28).

Once the cellular basis for vitamin D action could be assayed by in vitro estimation of $Ca^{+2}$ transport, many attempts were made to add the sterol directly to intestinal tissue, but these experiments showed no clear effect on calcium transport. When administered in vivo to vitamin-deficient rats, on the other hand, a distinct time lag was noted before the intestinal action could be observed. The systematic exploration of the significance of the time lag led De Luca and his colleagues (29, 30), Lawson and co-workers (31), and others to the discovery of the active metabolites of vitamin D. At least part of the time lag is required to convert vitamin D to active, hydroxylated products as described below. An additional important clue came from the demonstration that inhibitors of protein biosynthesis effectively block the action of the vitamin (32–34). Thus another reason for the obligatory time period before the onset of action of the vitamin is the requirement that proteins which are needed in the transport process be synthesized. These results led to direct approaches to the molecular basis of the calcium transport mechanism described above.

## MOLECULAR BASIS OF VITAMIN D ACTION

A simple scheme of the metabolism of vitamin D (calciferol, vitamin $D_2$; or cholecalciferol, vitamin $D_3$) is outlined in Figure 4. Sources are dietary vitamin $D_2$ or $D_3$, or endogenous $D_3$ formed by irradiation of 7-dehydrocholesterol in the skin. The sterol is hydroxylated to a more water-soluble product, 25-hydroxyvitamin D, in the liver, and this is in turn hydroxylated at the $C_1$ position in the kidney, with the formation of 1,25-

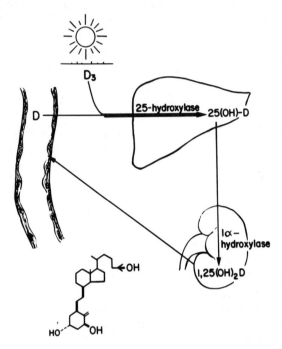

**Figure 4.** Major pathways in the activation (hydroxylation) of vitamin D from food sources or from the generation of vitamin $D_3$ in the skin. The structure of 1,25-dihydroxyvitamin D is shown.

dihydroxyvitamin D. The last compound is considerably more potent than the parent sterol, has a much decreased lag period, and appears to be the activated form of the sterol (30, 31) which acts on the enterocyte. The enzymatic hydroxylation in the kidney, via the enzyme $1\alpha$-hydroxylase, appears to be the rate limiting step in the overall sequence and as such is an important regulatory site. Two control loops shown in Figure 5 will illustrate the regulatory mechanisms. Increases in renal $1\alpha$-hydroxylase activity are stimulated by decreases in the concentration of plasma (extracellular) calcium or inorganic phosphate. Following the calcium control loop in Figure 5, a decrease in serum $Ca^{+2}$ stimulates release of parathormone, which increases renal $1\alpha$-hydroxylase activity. Enhanced synthesis of 1,25-dihydroxyvitamin D leads to increased intestinal absorption and, thereby, increased serum $Ca^{+2}$. Inasmuch as parathormone increases the urinary excretion of inorganic phosphate (Figure 5), the response to decreased serum $Ca^{+2}$ is relatively selective for the cation,

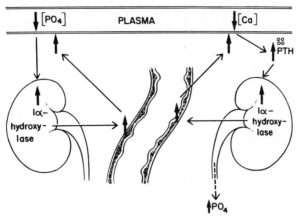

**Figure 5.** Regulatory loops in the control of calcium and phosphate absorption. Increases are signified by ↑ and decreases by ↓. See description in text.

that is, the accompanying stimulation of intestinal absorption of phosphate is counterbalanced. The second control loop in Figure 5 shows the regulatory response to decreased serum phosphate. Here the stimulus acts directly to increase the renal $1\alpha$-hydroxylase and the resulting enhanced synthesis of 1,25-dihydroxyvitamin D leads to increased intestinal absorption of inorganic phosphate and of calcium.

Further details of the action of 1,25-dihydroxyvitamin D on the enterocyte are illustrated in Figure 6. The active metabolite is bound to a specific carrier protein in the cytosol of the cell (35) and apparently acts at the level of the transcription of nuclear genes to elicit the synthesis of RNA coding for specific proteins required in the transport mechanisms.

## PROTEINS OF THE CALCIUM TRANSPORT MECHANISM

The search for vitamin D-dependent protein components of the calcium transport mechanism has been pursued energetically in a number of laboratories, for it may lead to an understanding of the molecular basis of the cation pump. To the present time two categories of mucosal proteins have been described. A soluble, calcium-binding protein (CaBP) was identified and characterized by Wasserman and co-workers (36–38) in chick mucosal homogenates, and similar proteins of relatively low molecular weight, approximately 12–24,000, have been observed in a number of species (39–41). While the CaBP activity of intestinal mucosa generally correlates with the level of calcium transport, some exceptions

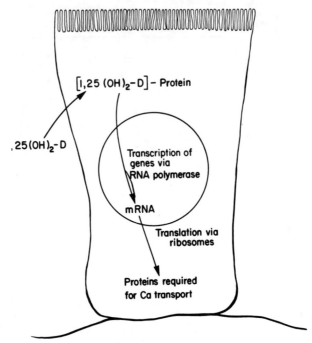

**Figure 6.** Action of 1,25-dihydroxyvitamin D in the intestinal enterocyte. See further description in the text.

have been noted, and it remains unclear how the soluble protein influences the transmembrane transit. The second type of mucosal component dependent on vitamin D is a particulate membrane fraction which was identified initially via its calcium-dependent adenosine triphosphatase (CaATPase) activity (42–45). My colleague, Szloma Kowarski, and I developed an isolation procedure for the particulate from rat intestinal mucosa and characterized it as a vitamin D-dependent complex which exhibits high affinity calcium binding as well as CaATPase and p-nitrophenylphosphatase activities (46). Our working hypothesis is that the particulate, named the Calcium-Binding Complex (CaBC), is the membrane protein mechanism for translocation of calcium.

To test the foregoing hypothesis the CaBC activity was correlated with known features of the calcium transport in rat intestine, and Figure 7 summarizes the results. Transport of calcium is dependent on vitamin D, greater in the duodenum as compared to the jejunum, greater in young, growing rats as compared to nongrowing, mature animals, greater in animals on a low calcium diet (0.02% Ca) as compared to a higher level

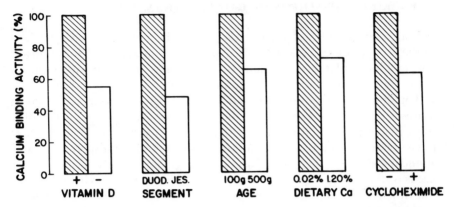

**Figure 7.** Effects of a number of biological variables on the Calcium-Binding Complex activity of rat intestinal mucosa. Calcium-binding activity was estimated as previously desribed (46) and a relative value (%) was calculated with reference to the control (higher) activity in each experiment.

diet (1.2% Ca), and inhibited by cycloheximide, which interferes with protein synthesis. As shown in Figure 7, the CaBC activity varies with each of these parameters as predicted from the corresponding effects on transport. Moreover, in an additional test we examined the effects of cycloheximide on the response of vitamin D-deficient rats to repletion. The compound very effectively blocked both the repair of the calcium transport mechanism and the CaBC activity.

Our efforts next turned to the solubilization, isolation, and characterization of the components of the CaBC. Rat CaBC can be solubilized by treatment with either 0.2% deoxycholate or n-butanol (47). The latter is now used routinely in our laboratory and yields extracts that are suitable for further purification. When the crude solubilized material which contains the three vitamin D-dependent activities, Ca binding, CaATPase, and p-nitrophenylphosphatase, is resolved by gel filtration on Sephadex G-150 followed by DEAE-cellulose anion exchange chromatography, the two enzyme activities co-elute with 0.1M NaCl, whereas the calcium-binding activity requires 0.3M NaCl for peak elution (48). The solubilized calcium-binding activity has now been purified further by hydroxylapatite gel chromatography to give a purified protein with an apparent molecular weight of approximately 200,000 as estimated by gel filtration chromatography. Biochemical and immunological studies are in progress to characterize the structure, cellular localization, and functions of this protein.

## A WORKING HYPOTHESIS OF CALCIUM TRANSPORT

It is apparent from the foregoing that only a beginning has been made in the attempt to unravel the molecular basis of intestinal calcium transport and its regulation by vitamin D. Nonetheless, it is heuristic to summarize our present understanding and to project a working model that will undoubtedly require modification as new findings emerge. Transmucosal transport of $Ca^{+2}$ across the enterocyte involves a sequence of steps, including entry at the microvillus (luminal) surface and exit across the basolateral membrane. The multistep nature of the transport and the abundant evidence that the absorption is regulated closely to meet the needs of the body for calcium make it highly likely that specific cellular constituents, probably membrane proteins or protein complexes, mediate the several transfer steps. The vitamin D action appears to be a regulatory mechanism developed in the course of evolution to facilitate the absorption of calcium needed for the skeleton and for locomotion. The sterol vitamin, following metabolic hydroxylation, influences specific protein biosynthetic processes in the enterocyte, apparently by eliciting specific mRNA synthesis. The proteins so encoded are required for maintenance of the active calcium pump mechanism and may well be integral parts of the pump machinery. The membrane-bound calcium-binding complex dependent on vitamin D may represent the calcium-translocating entity, particularly in the microvillus membrane (46). At such a luminal site, binding of a calcium ion to the calcium-binding component may be followed by translocation to the cytosol owing to the CaATPase (the p-nitrophenylphosphatase activity may be mediated by the CaATPase). The soluble CaBP of relatively low molecular weight may function as an intracellular carrier or as a regulator of cytosol calcium ion activity. Active transport of calcium out of the cell via the basolateral membrane may be mediated by an adenosine triphosphatase activity reported to be dependent on sodium and calcium (49).

Complex as the model above is, the truth will undoubtedly be even more complicated. Calcium is so important a body constituent and exhibits such powerful physiological and pharmacological actions that efficient regulation is mandatory. We can look forward to the discovery of additional entities and control processes. What a loss that Dan Kimberg will not share actively in the search—he would have loved it.

## REFERENCES

1. D. V. Kimberg, D. Schachter, and H. Schenker, *Am. J. Physiol.*, **200**, 1256 (1961)
2. D. Schachter, D. V. Kimberg, and H. Schenker, *Am. J. Physiol.*, **200**, 1263 (1961).

3. *Food and Nutrition Board: Recommended Dietary Allowances,* National Academy of Sciences-National Research Council, Washington, D.C., 1974, p. 86.

4. *FAO/WHO Expert Committee: Calcium Requirements,* WHO Tech. Report Ser. No. 1230, Geneva, 1962.

5. R. Nicolaysen, N. Eeg-Larsen, and O. J. Malm, *Physiol. Revs.,* **33,** 424 (1953).

6. L. Lack and I. M. Weiner, *Am. J. Physiol.,* **200,** 313 (1961).

7. S. Kowarski and D. Schachter, *J. Biol. Chem.* **244,** 211 (1969).

8. R. H. Wasserman and A. N. Taylor, *J. Nutr.,* **103,** 586 (1973).

9. A. N. Taylor, *J. Nutr.,* **104,** 489 (1974).

10. D. Schachter and S. M. Rosen, *Am. J. Physiol.,* **196,** 357 (1959).

11. D. Schachter, E. B. Dowdle, and H. Schenker, *Am. J. Physiol.,* **198,** 263 (1960).

12. E. B. Dowdle, D. Schachter, and H. Schenker, *Am. J. Physiol.,* **198,** 269 (1960).

13. H. Rasmussen, *Endocrinology,* **65,** 517 (1959).

14. H. E. Harrison and H. C. Harrison, *Am. J. Physiol.,* **199,** 265 (1960).

15. R. H. Wasserman, F. A. Kallfelz, and C. L. Comar, *Science,* **133,** 883 (1961).

16. D. Schachter, S. Kowarski, and P. Reid, in A. W. Cuthbert, Ed., *A Symposium on Calcium and Cellular Function,* Macmillan, London, 1969, p. 108.

17. D. Schachter, in R. M. Dowben, Ed., *Biological Membranes,* Little, Brown, Boston, 1969, p. 157.

18. D. Schachter, S. Kowarski, J. D. Finkelstein, and R.-I. W. Ma, *Am. J. Physiol.,* **211,** 1131 (1966).

19. W. Bloom and D. W. Fawcett, *A Textbook of Histology,* Saunders, Philadelphia, 1968, pp. 560-569.

20. Y. Okada, A. Irimajiri, and A. Inouye, *J. Membr. Biol.,* **31,** 221 (1977).

21. M. Fujita, K. Kawai, S. Asano, and M. Nakao, *Biochim. Biophys. Acta,* **307,** 141 (1973).

22. A. P. Douglas, R. Kerley, and K. J. Isselbacher, *Biochem. J.,* **128,** 1329 (1972).

23. H. Murer, U. Hopfer, E. Kinne-Saffran, and R. Kinne, *Biochim. Biophys. Acta,* **345,** 170 (1974).

24. T. A. Brasitus and D. Schachter, *Biochemistry,* manuscript submitted.

25. G. G. Forstner, K. Tanaka, and K. J. Isselbacher, *Biochem. J.* **109,** 51 (1968).

26. K. Kawai, M. Fujita, and M. Nakao, *Biochim. Biophys. Acta,* **369,** 222 (1974).

27. B. A. Lewis, G. M. Gray, R. Coleman, and R. H. Mitchell, *Biochem. Soc. Trans.,* **3,** 752 (1975).

28. R. A. Freedman, M. M. Weiser, and K. J. Issselbacher, *Proc. Natl. Acad. Sci. U.S.A.,* **74,** 3612 (1977).

29. J. W. Blunt, H. F. DeLuca, and H. K. Schnoes, *Biochemistry,* **7,** 3317 (1968).

30. M. F. Holick, H. K. Schnoes, and H. F. DeLuca, *Proc. Natl. Acad. Sci. U.S.A.,* **68,** 803 (1971).

31. D. E. Lawson, D. R. Fraser, E. Kodicek, H. R. Morris, and D. H. Williams, *Nature,* **230,** 228 (1971).

32. D. Schachter and S. Kowarski, *Bull. N.Y. Acad. Med.,* **41,** 241 (1965).

33. J. E. Zull, E. Czarnowski-Misztal, and H. F. DeLuca, *Science,* **149,** 182 (1965).

34. A. W. Norman, **149,** 184 (1965).

35. M. R. Haussler and T. A. McCain, *N. Engl. J. Med.,* **297,** 974 (1977).

36. R. H. Wasserman and A. N. Taylor, *Science,* **152,** 791 (1966).

37. R. H. Wasserman and A. N. Taylor, *J. Biol. Chem.,* **243,** 3987 (1968).

38. R. H. Wasserman, R. A. Corradino, and A. N. Taylor, *J. Biol. Chem.,* **243,** 3978 (1968).

39. D. H. Alpers, S. W. Lee, and L. V. Avioli, *Gastroenterology,* **62,** 559 (1972).

40. D. Schachter, S. Kowarski, and P. Reid, *J. Clin. Invest.,* **46,** 113a (1967).

41. C. S. Fullmer and R. H. Wasserman, *Biochim. Biophys. Acta,* **317,** 172 (1973).

42. D. L. Martin, M. J. Melancon, Jr., and H. F. DeLuca, *Biochem. Biophys. Res. Commun.,* **35,** 89 (1969).

43. M. J. Melancon, Jr. and H. F. DeLuca, *Biochemistry,* **9,** 1658 (1970).

44. M. R. Haussler, L. A. Nagode, and H. Rasmussen, *Nature,* **228,** 1199 (1970).

45. S. Kowarski and D. Schachter, *J. Clin Invest.,* **52,** 2765 (1973).

46. S. Kowarski and D. Schachter, *Am. J. Physiol.,* **229,** 1198 (1975).

47. S. Kowarski and D. Schachter, *Fed. Proc.,* **36,** 510 (1977).

48. D. Schachter and S. Kowarski, in C. Anast and H. F. DeLuca, Eds., *Pediatric Diseases Related to Calcium,* Elsevier, New York, 1979, in press.

49. S. J. Birge, H. R. Gilbert, and L. V. Avioli, *Science,* **176,** 168 (1972).

# PART 2

# Gastrointestinal Diseases that Affect Nutrition

# 6

## Malabsorption Syndromes Including Disease of Pancreatic and Biliary Origin

KURT J. ISSELBACHER, M.D.

Massachusetts General Hospital, Harvard Medical School, Boston, Massachusetts

When one is confronted with a clinical problem of malabsorption, one must determine whether the patient simply has diarrhea with excessive fluid and nutrient loss, in which malabsorption is secondary, or whether the malabsorption is primary, with diarrhea a secondary manifestation. Thus, the way that the individual patient presents determines whether the initial workup should be for the diarrhea, for malabsorption, or for both. Therefore I shall initially consider just the mechanism involved in the production of diarrhea.

Increase in fluid in the intestine as it leaves the colon may be due in part to a net balance of *increased secretion* (1). Fluid may shift as a result of increased osmotic activity in the lumen or enhanced motility may be contributing to the rate at which nutrients move through the intestinal tract. As a result these nutrients may not be absorbed adequately. Table 1 is a list of the secretory diarrheas. Mechanisms for increasing secretion that may be associated with an adenylate cyclase increase, an area to which Dr. Kimberg actively contributed, demonstrate that a variety of endogenous and exogenous agents may produce diarrhea, increasing secretion by stimulating this enzyme in the intestinal cell. Such agents include exogenous toxins, endogenous agents, such as prostaglandins, or various hormonally active peptides, bile acids, and so on. There can also be secretion that apparently does not involve this enzyme system, such as that induced by certain laxatives, other bacterial enterotoxins, and hormones. The third mechanism whereby the intestine can secrete is as a result of mucosal injury and altered cell permeability,

Table 1    Secretory Mechanisms in the Production of Diarrhea

1. Secretion associated with ↑ adenylate cyclase
   a. Enterotoxins (V. cholera; E. coli)
   b. Prostaglandins
   c. Vasoactive intestinal peptide (VIP)
   d. Bile acids (dihydroxy); affect colon primarily
2. Secretion with no effect on adenylate cyclase
   a. Laxatives (ricinoleic acid, phenolphthalein)
   b. Bacterial enterotoxins (shigella, staph aureus)
   c. Hormones, peptides (glucagon, secretin, serotonin, calcitonin, GIP)
3. Mucosal injury, altered cell permeability
   a. Invasive microorganism (salmonella, shigella, certain E. coli, and viruses)
   b. Inflammatory bowel disease
   c. Sprue
4. Neoplasms (often with hormone production)

such as that produced by infections, microorganisms, inflammatory bowel disease, and sprue. Neoplasms may or may not be associated with increased hormone production. *Osmotic* effects include impaired carbohydrate absorption, such as the disaccharidase deficiency syndromes, and increasing fluid shifts as a result of laxatives that increase the osmotic activity in the intestinal lumen. Finally there are other derangements of motility, where laxatives, instead of producing osmotic changes, stimulate bowel contractility; changes in bowel function that appear to be components of the irritable bowel syndrome; derangements that may be seen with diverticular disease of the colon; and diabetic diarrhea, where neurologic changes involving the visceral nerves may contribute to derangements in motility. This represents only a partial list of the disorders that may produce diarrhea. Some may be associated with malabsorption and this must be considered in approaching the overall problem.

## MALABSORPTION

In considering a patient with the possibility of malabsorption, I prefer first to determine whether the process may be intraluminal and hence a problem of maldigestion rather than one primarily involving the cell per se. One area that would fall into this category of impaired or inadequate digestion is *postgastrectomy states*. We do not know the overall mechanism, but we know factors that contribute to the impaired digestion in such instances, such as inadequate mixing of nutrients when they are digested. A second area is *pancreatic insufficiency*. Pancreatic enzymes are needed to carry out intraluminal disgestion and it is evident that the pH is very important; hence, the amount of bicarbonate secreted by the pancreas to neutralize the acid of the stomach and to create a pH above 6, which would be favorable for pancreatic enzyme digestion, is important. Although major pancreatic enzyme deficiency must be present before evidence of pancreatic insufficiency becomes clinically apparent, the pancreas is extremely important in this overall intraluminal process. The pH is particularly important as emphasized by the findings in the Zollinger-Ellison syndrome in which there is a so-called gastrinoma, or gastrin-producing tumor, found in the pancreas, with excessive production of acid and a resulting malabsorption primarily due to changes in pH. Another consideration involves our natural detergents, the bile salts. If these are not adequate in amount to permit proper micelle formation there may not be either adequate hydrolysis or lypolysis of the lipid that is ingested, or these lipids may not be adequately presented to the intestinal cell for transport.

## CONDITIONS REFLECTING DERANGEMENTS AT THE CELLULAR LEVEL

First we must consider a reduction in the absorbing surface, as occurs with extensive resection of small intestine. Second, we may see this reduction in patients with generalized inflammatory bowel disease; this disorder tends usually not to involve the upper small intestine but certainly involves the ileum. Hence disorders with impaired ileal absorption are important. If there is insufficient oxygenation of the mucosa, due either to venous or to arterial insufficiency, one may see a typical malabsorption state. Bacterial overgrowth in the small intestine, as with stasis and blind loops, may cause impaired absorption. If the outflow from the intestinal cells into the lymphatics is obstructed by tumor or congenital obstruction of the thoracic duct, there may be not only congestion of the mucosa but also impaired absorption, especially of lipid. Finally, specific cellular disorders where the mucosal cell per se seems to be altered may result in malabsorption.

## Sprue

The prototype of malabsorption is sprue, a disease that has been studied for many years (2). During the last 30 years we have gathered a reasonable amount of information but we still lack some important details. At first, sprue went under a variety of names. As a way of distinguishing it from tropical sprue, the term nontropical sprue was used. The similarity to what was found in pediatric celiac disease or adult celiac disease, depending on the age, created some confusion. The determination that gluten, the protein in wheat, played a role in this syndrome resulted in the term gluten-induced enteropathy. The result is that there is a component of this protein which, in the affected individual, leads to deleterious changes in the mucosa resulting in impaired absorption of many nutrients. The major clinical features are not really specific—they simply reflect what may happen in anyone with significant malabsorption. By definition, diarrhea and steatorrhea (the increased loss of fat) are the hallmarks of impaired absorption. The stools are malodorous, in part due to the increased fat in the form of short-chain fatty acids. These acids, in addition, may result in abdominal disteniton due to an increased amount of gas in the intestinal lumen. The weight loss due to malnutrition obviously reflects the degree of impaired absorption as does the hypoalbuminemia that will develop if the malabsorption is pronounced. The anemia may be of various types because the patient may have a deficiency in the absorption of vitamin $B_{12}$ or iron or folate; the nature of the anemia depends upon which of these predominates. It is only in the severe case that symptoms such as tetany or changes in bone will occur as a result of the pronounced impairment in the absorption of calcium or vitamin D. Similarly it is not too common to see patients with reductions in circulating prothrombin levels due to the impaired absorption of vitamin K. Although many or all of these changes may occur, there are many patients with atypical presentations; thus we may find only some of these components present clinically or by laboratory examination.

One way to diagnose sprue or gluten-induced enteropathy is by intestinal biopsy. The term "villous atrophy" has been used because the villi appear minimal or absent under the dissecting microscope. Even to the naked eye the mucosa looks flat instead of having its normal fingerlike appearance. However, this is really not "atrophy" because there is actually an increased synthesis of crypt cells. Nevertheless, the result is that differentiation of crypt cells to mature villus cells is inadequate; as a result the surface appears flat. Thus there is an increase in the crypt: villus cell ratio. It should be emphasized that crypt cells, in contrast to the mature villi, have a reduced absorptive capacity. They are still immature and undifferentiated and have not yet geared up to carry out all of the transport function. Hence, if the intestine is populated with an abundance of crypt cells, there may be an adequate number of cells but not an adequate number of those that have differentiated sufficiently to carry out maximum absorptive function. In addition, there are other morphologic changes. The villus cells that are present often seem to be more cuboidal and columnar and to have derangements, so that we have both an increase in crypt cells and a change in the villus cells—both features contributing to impaired absorption. In addition there is a cellular infiltration of the lamina propria. Thus we can make a diagnosis that is "consistent with sprue" by intestinal biopsy. When one finds a biopsy with the above morphologic changes, the patient should be placed on a gluten-free diet. We would then expect clinical as well as morphologic improvement. This may occur within a matter of days or certainly weeks, and often can be very dramatic. We recognize, however, that whatever the underlying defect, it will persist, since if the patient is reexposed to the offending agent, both malabsorption and the morphologic changes will recur. What remains to be answered is how gluten produces its deleterious effects in patients with sprue.

There are some data that do reflect on this problem. A number of years ago it was shown that when gluten was deaminated, so that the terminal amino group of the glutamine was removed, the protein lost its toxicity when fed to patients with sprue. In addition, if gluten was broken down to polypeptides it could be demonstrated that the larger peptides induced steatorrhea in patients with sprue. However, if this hydrolysis was carried out thoroughly either to individual amino acids or to peptides less than eight amino acids in number, the toxicity was lost. Thus it is attractive to speculate that, either on a familial or possibly on an acquired basis, patients may have a deficiency of a certain peptidase. But given the number of amino acids involved and hence the number of combinations of these amino acids, to determine which peptidase might be deficient is a real problem. Hence this hypothesis remains a possibility but it is one that has not been clearly demonstrated.

A peptidase deficiency could be combined with some of the immunologic derangements that have been observed in sprue. In recent years studies have demonstrated an increase in immunoglobulin synthesis in the intestine (especially IgM). Increased levels of IgA are found in the serum. Whether these immunologic changes are primary or secondary is not clear. In addition, patients with sprue tend to have a greater incidence of the genetic marker HLA-B8, suggesting that genetic factors make certain individuals more susceptible to developing sprue than others. The available data suggest to me that a specific deficiency of a peptidase may result in an incomplete breakdown of gluten, leading to a "toxic peptide" that could produce cell damage, which in turn can lead to the immunologic changes that have been described. Another possibility, although a less likely one in my judgment, is that there is an underlying and primary immunologic disorder which is triggered by gluten. Whatever the mechanism, malabsorption may be due to villous cell damage, to increase in crypt cells, or to both; both of these changes will decrease absorption by the small intestine.

A third criterion for establishing the diagnosis of sprue, using the organ culture technique, has recently been introduced. A sprue biopsy put in organ culture and exposed to gluten will have a diminished synthesis of enzymes such as alkaline phosphatase. This observation is provocative and obviously will need to be pursued. Will such a change in enzyme synthesis still be evident in the patient after he has been on a gluten-free diet say for a year or two? Data to answer this question are not yet available. Once the diagnosis has been made and a gluten-free diet prescribed, what must one consider if the patient does not improve? First, the diet may not have been strict enough. Second, when one is dealing with a damaged mucosa, lactase deficiency will usually also be present and hence, if milk is in the diet, the patient may still have symptoms due to the ingestion of lactose. Third, certain patients may develop carcinoma or lymphoma of the small intestine. Finally, one must question whether the diagnosis may not be correct, since at present we have no specific diagnostic tests for sprue.

### Impaired Carbohydrate Absorption

We next consider impaired absorption of carbohydrates (both monosaccharides and disaccharides). The most common of these is lactase deficiency. Deficiencies of sucrase and maltase seem less common, but I suspect that with some of the newer techniques available, we will find that there are more patients with either an acquired or a hereditary impairment of this particular enzyme system than we have suspected.

There is a very high incidence of reduced lactase activity in certain segments of the population of the world, especially in Orientals and blacks, where the incidence can be as high as 80 to 90%. Individuals with lactase deficiency will develop diarrhea and abdominal distention after lactose ingestion. One can diagnose the disorder clinically either on the basis of a history or by the clinical changes following lactose administration. An oral lactose tolerance test will show an impaired rise in blood sugar after the ingestion of 50 to 100 g of lactose. The diagnosis can also be made by measuring breath hydrogen (3). Patients will show an increase in breath hydrogen after ingesting lactose. Lactose acts as a laxative because it is not hydrolyzed; the unabsorbed lactose then exerts osmotic effects leading to a shifting of fluid into the intestinal lumen. If enough lactose gets into the lower small intestine or colon it will be hydrolyzed by bacteria. The lactic acid and hydrogen so produced provide the basis of the breath test, and also lead to abdominal distention and gas. Often the symptoms occur so promptly that one wonders how much the production of lactic acid has to do with the symptoms. One of the features that has been puzzling pediatricians is the age of appearance of lactase deficiency. Most studies indicate that the deficiency becomes evident around age five to eight, depending on the particular population under study. It is clear that during gestation enzyme activity is low but then rises and is highest shortly after birth. There is then a gradual decline in intestinal lactase activity. It would seem that those with lactose intolerance may have a lower level at birth, and by eight to twelve years of age their enzyme levels will be much lower than normal. How much of a decrease of lactase is needed to become symptomatic? The answer is not clear.

The breath hydrogen test is based on the concept that normally sugars such as lactose are hydrolyzed and very little of the sugar is left to be acted upon by bacteria. Hence the amount of hydrogen absorbed from the colon and present in the respiratory air is very low. On the other hand, when one ingests a sugar, such as lactulose, which is normally not hydrolyzed but can be metabolized by bacteria, an abundance of hydrogen will be produced and appear in increased amounts in the breath (3). The hydrogen can be measured readily with various gas chromatographic techniques. The amount of hydrogen exhaled seems to be proportional to the amount of hydrogen produced in the colon. For hydrogen to be produced in increased amounts two components are required—bacteria and a fermentable nutrient. The appearance of breath hydrogen can be used not only to detect malabsorption but also to quantitate the magnitude of the problem. As with any technique, there can be false positives and false negatives and it is quite likely that as the technique is employed more extensively we will learn more about the limits of this method. For example, if we had bacterial overgrowth we might get a false positive result. With rapid intestinal motility one might get a false negative because the nutrient moves so rapidly through the intestinal tract that there is not sufficient time for bacteria to produce the hydrogen. If the patient has been on antibiotics and the intestinal flora has been reduced one might also get a negative result. But these problems usually can be detected and I mention them because undoubtedly as

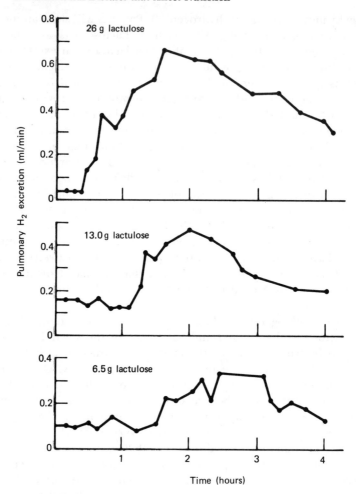

**Figure 1.** Breath hydrogen after varying doses of lactulose [from Bond and Levitt (3)].

this test is employed with increasing frequency these false positive and negative values will assume more significance. Figure 1, taken from the work of Bond and Levitt (3), shows how increasing the amount of lactulose, which is not hydrolyzed but is metabolized by bacteria, will lead to an increase in pulmonary or breath hydrogen excretion. Thus the increase in breath hydrogen correlates with the amount of lactulose administered. Normally this increase in hydrogen excretion begins at about 1 hour and peaks at about 2 or 3 hours after the ingestion of lactulose. The breath hydrogen technique is no longer as complicated as it was and simple techniques whereby air is aspirated from the nose or the

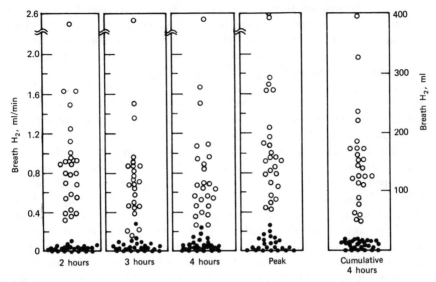

**Figure 2.** Breath hydrogen after lactose in normal subjects (black dots) and patients with lactase deficiency (open circles).

pharynx are as effective as the more complicated procedures. Figure 2 is an example of the breath hydrogen in normals compared to patients with lactase deficiency.

Determinations of breath hydrogen changes can be performed with any sugar or any nutrient. We have done these experiments successfully with amino acids in rats and I am optimistic that this kind of approach will permit us to detect other disorders that to date may have been considered functional or psychosomatic. Using this technique with sucrose ingestion, we have discovered patients with sucrose intolerance.

Tropical sprue differs from the gluten-induced enteropathy. It seems to be a reflection and consequence of an altered gut flora. The nature of this flora and what there is about it that induces the morphologic changes and derangements in folic acid metabolism are still subject to debate. It was recently suggested that certain types of E. coli may predominate in this disease. Tropical sprue is usually correctable with broad spectrum antibiotics, folic acid, or both.

### Ileal Disease

The ileum is important for the absorption of $B_{12}$ and of bile salts. Certain disorders may be the result of impairment in bile salt reabsorption, leading to an increased loss of bile salts in the stool. In addition to diarrhea and steatorrhea ileal resection may lead to increased oxalate absorption, with an increased oxalate in the urine and hence renal stone formation. In the normal enterohepatic circulation, the bile salts are produced by the liver and excreted into the duodenum, and 95% of the bile salts are reabsorbed in the ileum. Therefore only small amounts (0.3 to 0.6 g/day) are excreted in the stool. An increase in bile salts in the stool can lead to an increased fluid loss and diarrhea. Bile salts have a laxative effect because when they reach the colon in excessive amounts they can produce secretion of electrolytes and water. This effect is correctable if we bind the bile salts with a sequestrant such as cholestyramine; thus, although they are present in the colon in increased amounts, they are prevented from exerting their effect on the mucosa. If the bile salt loss is too extensive, the liver may not be able to keep up with the loss and the intraluminal bile salts levels become too low. As a result one may see both steatorrhea and diarrhea. Therapeutically this state of affairs is difficult to treat because if we give cholestyramine we will bind and excrete more bile salts, which will not help to correct the intraluminal bile salt concentration in the small intestine. One may need to resort to the use of medium-chain triglycerides, which do not require a high micellar concentration of bile salts in order to be absorbed. In summary, an increased concentration of bile salts in the colon stimulates colonic adenylate cyclase, leading to an impairment in the absorption of electrolytes and water and to some extent also in the net secretion of electrolytes and water. If the bile salt loss is not extensive the liver is able to compensate by producing more bile salts so that the luminal concentration of bile salts can be maintained. If this loss is extensive, the intraluminal levels are not sufficient for micelle formation and one may develop an increased fat loss in addition to fluid loss. One of the problems in patients with ileal resection or disease is oxaluria. How does this occur? A patient with an ileostomy will generally not develop increased oxalate in the urine because it has been shown that the oxalate must reach the colon, where it is then absorbed. When there is an increased amount of fat in the intestinal lumen, the normal amount of calcium which we would like to be available to produce insoluble calcium oxalate is instead bound to fatty acids to form insoluble calcium salts of fatty acids. As a result, there is not sufficient calcium left to form calcium oxalate and in turn the free oxalate can be absorbed. In addition to there being more free oxalate there is a change in colonic permeability to oxalate in patients with an increased amount of fatty acids or bile acids in the colonic lumen. Thus two factors contribute: increasing amounts of free oxalate reaching the colon and an altered permeability permitting greater uptake of oxalate at that site. One can correct this phenomenon by decreasing the dietary intake of oxalate or by giving more oral calcium, magnesium, or aluminum salts. Cholestyramine also seems to work but the mechanism of its action is not clear. One theory is that it prevents the effect of the bile acids on colonic permeability; however, the evidence for this mechanism is not yet conclusive. Finally, gallstone formation is increased with ileal disease because bile acids are lost in significant amounts. As a result the bile acids in the bile duct and gallbladder are reduced and this tends to make the bile lithogenic and permits cholesterol to come out of solution.

## Malabsorption due to Bacterial Overgrowth

Any condition in the small intestine that leads to stasis will permit the proliferation of bacteria. Such bacterial overgrowth may lead to impaired absorption of $B_{12}$ (because of increased utilization of $B_{12}$ by the bacteria), steatorrhea, diarrhea, or disaccharidase deficiency. In rats it has been shown that bacterial proteases in the small intestine may remove some of the surface enzymes (including the disaccharidases) and produce disaccharidase deficiency. Several mechanisms have been proposed to explain the malabsorption. First, the bacteria can hydrolyze the conjugated bile salts resulting in decreased micelle formation because of a decreased conjugated bile salt concentration; the result is increased fat in the stool. The bacterial conversion of bile salts to deoxycholic acid is enhanced. Deoxycholate is a very potent stimulus of adenylate cyclase and enhances colonic cyclic AMP formation—a mechanism that can produce diarrhea. Finally, bacteria can convert fatty acids to more potent laxative agents such as hydroxy fatty acids. The effect of castor oil on the intestine is a typical example of the laxative action of hydroxy fatty acids. To make the diagnosis of bacterial overgrowth one can obviously try to demonstrate the increase in bacteria by aspiration and colony counts. In the absence of this direct evidence one may use antibiotics and observe whether the clinical or laboratory parameters are altered. A technique that was used in the past but is not used as frequently now is to measure the production of a certain bacterial metabolite, such as indican; indicanuria is increased in patients with bacterial overgrowth. Finally, one may use the technique of using a labeled radioactive glycocholate (with the glycine labeled). Gut bacteria will remove the labeled glycine from the glycocholate; the glycine then is absorbed and goes to the liver to be converted to $CO_2$. The latter is then exhaled and recovered in the respiratory air, where it can be collected and measured.

We have reviewed some of the important disorders leading to malabsorption. Although there are others, those reviewed are perhaps the most common. In any event I hope that this discussion will provide a reasonable insight into the current views about these disorders and the techniques that have promise in studying and diagnosing the various malabsorption states.

## REFERENCES

1. M. Field, Intestinal secretion, *Gastroenterology*, **66,** 1063 (1974).
2. N. J. Greenberger and K. J. Isselbacher, "Disorders of Absorption and Malabsorption," *in* Harrison's *Principles of Internal Medicine*, 9th ed., McGraw-Hill, New York, 1980.
3. J. H. Bond and M. D. Levitt, Use of hydrogen ($H_2$) in the study of carbohydrate absorption, *Am. J. Digest. Dis.*, **22,** 379 (1977).

# 7

# Malabsorption of Vitamin $B_{12}$ and Folate

Columbia University, College of Physicians and Surgeons, Harlem Hospital Center, New York, New York

## VITAMIN $B_{12}$ ABSORPTION

### Cobalamins in Food

Vitamin $B_{12}$ (cobalamin; Cbl) is found almost exclusively in foods containing animal protein (1), although certain seaweeds (2) and well water contaminated with enteric bacteria (3) may serve as unusual sources of cobalamin. Because of the extensive storage of cobalamins in the body, strict vegetarianism for prolonged periods of time is required for the development of true nutritional $B_{12}$ deficiency in an adult. Therefore, in the United States at least, in virtually all patients who develop significant cobalamin deficiency, a disturbance in the pathways for absorption of the vitamin can be demonstrated.

Deoxyadenosyl-Cbl and hydroxo-Cbl are the predominant coenzyme forms present in most foods of animal origin, although lesser amounts of methyl-Cbl, sulfito-Cbl, or cyano-Cbl (CN-Cbl) may be present in certain foods (4). In human subjects, purified CN-Cbl and hydroxo-Cbl appear to be more or less equally well absorbed; deoxyadenosyl-Cbl, methyl-Cbl, and sulfito-Cbl are less well assimilated (4, 5). Some cobalamin may be destroyed during prolonged boiling or broiling of foods (6). The absorption in normal subjects of foods containing radiolabeled cobalamins has been studied by several groups of investigators. Vitamin $B_{12}$ in chicken meat and mutton were absorbed as well as crystalline CN-Cbl, whereas that in eggs was poorly absorbed, in part because of an inhibitor of cobalamin absorption in ovalbumin (6–10).

Vitamin $B_{12}$ in foods is bound to protein, although the exact nature of the binding proteins remains to be elucidated. In order for food cobalamins to be absorbed, these bonds must be broken and the cobalamin ultimately transferred to intrinsic factor in the gastrointestinal lumen. Although published in vitro studies have shown conflicting results, most observers have found that a certain amount of liberation of food $B_{12}$ into a dialyzable form may occur at neutral pH during the process of homogenization or cooking, with further generation of free $B_{12}$ at low pH, with or without added pepsin (11–14). The relative importance of cooking, acid, and pepsin remains to be established, and probably varies depending on the individual food (11–14).

## Role of the Stomach

In recent years, a number of investigators have called attention to a subtle form of $B_{12}$ malabsorption, in which cobalamin deficiency is believed to have developed as a result of inability to liberate cobalamins from food in the presence of adequate amounts of intrinsic factor. This may occur in patients who have had a partial gastrectomy, or a vagotomy with gastroenterostomy, or who have chronic gastritis with achlorhydria or hypochlorhydria (7, 8, 10, 15–19). In most instances, low serum $B_{12}$ concentrations have been noted despite the presence of a normal Schilling test performed with crystalline CN-Cbl. When these patients were given radiolabeled Cbl incorporated into eggs or chicken meat, or CN-Cbl bound in vitro to ovalbumin or chicken serum, absorption of these protein-bound cobalamin preparations was subnormal. These observations appear to establish an entity of food cobalamin malabsorption due to lack of acid, lack of pepsin, or both. It should be noted, however, that most of these patients have decreased, although not markedly diminished, intrinsic factor secretion, and CN-Cbl absorption by standard Schilling tests may be intermittently subnormal (20). Furthermore, whereas low serum $B_{12}$ levels are not unusual in these patients, the development of frank $B_{12}$ deficiency is relatively rare, and when it occurs is often associated with other factors that cause a negative balance of cobalamins, such as poor dietary intake, or D. latum infestation (18, 21). These clinical observations are consistent with the in vitro findings of several workers, which indicate that a certain fraction of food $B_{12}$ becomes dialyzable even without the addition of acid or pepsin (12, 14). Thus, it is likely that any requirement for acid–peptic digestion of food cobalamin–protein bonds is only partial and will apply only to a fraction of the dietary vitamin sources. The requirement for intrinsic factor is absolute, and is sensitively assayed by the routine Schilling test. Thus, virtu-

**Table 1   Vitamin B$_{12}$-Binding Proteins**

| Protein | Origin | Fluid | Mol. Wt | Nature | Function |
|---|---|---|---|---|---|
| Intrinsic factor | Parietal cell | Gastric juice | 44,000 | Glycoprotein | Deliver dietary B$_{12}$ to ileum |
| Transcobalamin II | Liver, ? gut | Serum | 38,000 | Polypeptide | Transport B$_{12}$ from gut, deliver B$_{12}$ to cells |
| R-binders (including transcobalamins I and III) | Many cells (including granulo-cytes) | Serum, bile milk, saliva, gastric juice | 58,000–66,000 | Glycoprotein | Transport B$_{12}$ and analogs to liver, ? rid body of analogs, ? antibacterial |

ally all patients who develop clinically significant B$_{12}$ deficiency related to atrophic gastritis or partial gastrectomy will have abnormal absorption of CN-Cbl (22, 23).

Once cobalamins are liberated from food, they must become bound (sooner or later) to intrinsic factor (Table 1) in order for ileal uptake and absorption to occur. Intrinsic factor deficiency occurs most frequently as a result of severe chronic atrophic gastritis ("pernicious anemia") or following partial or total gastrectomy (22, 23). In patients with pernicious anemia the main cause of cobalamin depletion is lack of intrinsic factor, although binding of intrinsic factor by intraluminal antibodies, bacterial overgrowth secondary to achlorhydria, and reversible ileal dysfunction due to B$_{12}$ deficiency itself may contribute to malabsorption of the vitamin (24, 50). Rarely, B$_{12}$ lack occurs early in childhood in patients with an apparent isolated inherited defect in intrinsic factor synthesis, in association with an otherwise normal stomach which secretes abundant hydrochloric acid (so-called "congenital pernicious anemia") (25). Of great theoretical interest was the recent report of a child who developed cobalamin deficiency as a result of the secretion of an abnormal intrinsic factor that was able to bind B$_{12}$ well but had markedly decreased ability to promote cobalamin uptake by ileal homogenates (26). Such a disorder has not yet been described on an acquired basis.

## ROLE OF THE PANCREAS

As a result of the elegant studies of Allen and co-workers, it is now realized that substantial amounts of dietary cobalamins may be bound in the gastrointestinal lumen, at least transiently, to so-called R-binders (see Table 1) present in saliva, gastric juice, bile, and intestinal juices (27, 28). At low pH, R-binders have a much greater affinity for cobalamins than intrinsic factor, and virtually all $B_{12}$ added to an equimolar mixture of the two binders in purified form at pH 2 will be bound to the R-binder (28). Even at pH 8, two to three times as much cobalamin will be bound to the R-binder. Since R-binders do not promote ileal uptake of the vitamin, if gastrointestinal fluids were no more than a simplified mixture of these binders and dietary cobalamins, most of the $B_{12}$ in an oral dose would not be absorbed (which is not the case in vivo). Allen and co-workers have shown that pancreatic proteases partially degrade R-binders in vitro and allow $B_{12}$ to be transferred with time to intrinsic factor (28).

That a similar situation may occur in the gastrointestinal tract may be argued from the finding that approximately 50% of patients with pancreatic insufficiency absorb CN-Cbl poorly, and that this malabsorption may be completely corrected by pancreatic enzyme preparations or by purified trypsin, and partially corrected by bicarbonate administration (29–32). Further, the administration of a $B_{12}$ analog in amounts large enough to saturate gastrointestinal R-binders normalized CN-Cbl absorption in patients with pancreatic insufficiency (33).

Other observations, however, call into question the absolute requirement for pancreatic proteases in cobalamin absorption in humans. Some patients who have undergone total pancreatectomy may have normal CN-Cbl absorption (31, 34). In addition, in some individuals with pancreatic insufficiency and abnormal Schilling tests, CN-Cbl absorption is normalized when the radioactive $B_{12}$ is given with a meal (33, 35). Finally, and most persuasively, cobalamin deficiency is extremely unusual (or does not occur) in patients with pancreatic insufficiency in the absence of other disturbances in cobalamin absorption, such as pernicious anemia. These observations suggest that even in the absence of pancreatic enzymes, enough dietary cobalamin is transferred to intrinsic factor to prevent the depletion of body stores. One important factor may be the location in the gastrointestinal tract where food $B_{12}$ is transferred to the various binders (which is unknown). If much of this occurred in the small bowel rather than the stomach, and therefore at a higher pH, substantial cobalamin binding by intrinsic factor might occur. Studies in vivo of the actual luminal events in the processing of food cobalamins will undoubtedly be performed in the next decade to clarify these questions. In an in vivo study using an oral dose of CN-Cbl given in the fasting state to normal subjects as well as patients with tropical sprue, 37 to 75% of the radioactive $B_{12}$ was found to be bound to intrinsic factor in the first loop of jejunum (36).


## INTESTINAL BACTERIA

In the blind loop syndrome, or in infestation with the fish tapeworm, D. latum, overgrowth of the jejunum with bacteria or the parasite leads to cobalimin deficiency (22). In both these situations the offending organisms have been shown to bind and internalize vitamin $B_{12}$ even if it is bound to gastric juice. Bacterial overgrowth is most commonly encountered clinically in patients with multiple jejunal diverticulae or following gastrointestinal surgery. Many species of enteric bacteria rapidly bind cobalamin in vitro in a first step that appears to be adsorption to a surface receptor, followed by a second step involving cobalamin transport to the interior of the cell (37, 38). The interaction of these organisms with $B_{12}$ bound to purified intrinsic factor and R-binder has not yet been studied. In addition to robbing the host of cobalamin, enteric bacteria may convert the vitamin to various absorbable or nonabsorbable analogs, which may compete for binding sites on intrinsic factor and therefore further impair $B_{12}$ absorption (39).


## ILEAL EVENTS

Cobalamins are present in high concentration in bile, probably bound to R-binders (27). While it has often been assumed that there is an extensive enterophepatic circulation, the percentage of biliary $B_{12}$ that is reabsorbed in the ileum is unknown.

Since the ileum is the main site of active $B_{12}$ absorption from the vitamin concentrations present in food (although passive absorption of cobalamins given in massive doses may occur throughout the small bowel), any disorder involving the ileum may lead to deficiency. Relatively common examples include ileal resection, regional enteritis, tropical sprue, and celiac disease (22). In tropical sprue, bacterial overgrowth may contribute to $B_{12}$ malabsorption in many cases, and (less commonly) an associated gastritis may markedly impair intrinsic factor secretion (40).

Understanding of the events occurring in the ileum during cobalamin transport into the portal venous system remains limited. The presence of a microvillus receptor site for the $B_{12}$–intrinsic factor complex has been well demonstrated, as has the pH and calcium dependence of this step, which involves a nonenergy-requiring attachment to a membrane protein (22, 40a, 40b, 41). The receptor protein has been solubilized and a number of investigators have recently reported its purification by affinity chromatography (41a–41c). Receptor activity has been found throughout the distal three-fifths of the human small bowel; it is maximal just before the terminal ileum (42). A delay of several hours takes place during the uphill transport of cobalamin across the ileal cell, which occurs against a concentration gradient (as in the Schilling test). It is likely that the $B_{12}$–intrinsic factor complex is internalized by the ileal enterocyte (42a, 42b). In animals, the vitamin is transiently associated with mitochondria during the delay period in the ileal cell (43). Cobalamin emerges from the intestine and is found in the portal circulation bound to transcobalamin II; intrinsic factor does not enter the portal blood (22, 27, 44). There is increasing evidence that transcobalamin II is required for absorption to occur, and that the vitamin may be bound to this protein before it emerges from the ileal cell (44–44b). Of the three families reported with congenital transcobalamin II deficiency, three patients have been studied and all have been found to malabsorb vitamin $B_{12}$ (45–47). Rigorous proof that this binder is essential for cobalamin absorption, or that it is synthesized by ileal cells, is lacking, however.

Which of the various ileal steps in $B_{12}$ assimilation is interrupted by various disease states is obscure. In the single patient with hereditary selective $B_{12}$ malabsorption that has been studied to date, the binding activity of the ileal receptor site for the $B_{12}$–intrinsic factor complex was found to be normal (48).

Cobalamin deficiency itself may cause a morphologically "megaloblastic" gut, which reverts to normal after vitamin therapy (49). In three-quarters of patients with pernicious anemia, the deficiency state was associated with malabsorption of CN-Cbl given with intrinsic factor (50). Intrinsic factor-mediated cobalamin absorption usually returned to normal within 1 to 8 weeks of treatment with the vitamin (50).

Therapy with a number of drugs, including para-amino salicyclic acid, neomycin, colchicine, and biguanides (51–54), as well as chronic intoxication with alcohol (55), may cause cobalamin malabsorption, presumably at the ileal level. However, the development of clinically significant deficiency as a result of ingestion of any of these agents has not been reported.

Massive hypersecretion of acid caused by a gastrin-producing tumor (the Zollinger-Ellison syndrome) may be associated with $B_{12}$ malabsorption which is correctable by bicarbonate administration. The exact mechanism is unknown (56), but possible explanations could invoke im-

Table 2    Cause of Cobalamin Deficiency in 123 Consecutive Cases of Megaloblastic Anemia in New York City[a]

|  | Number of Cases | |
| --- | --- | --- |
| Pernicious anemia[b] | 87 | (70.7%) |
| Partial or total gastrectomy | 4 | (3.3%) |
| Multiple jejunal diverticulae | 5 | (4.1%) |
| Tropical sprue[c] | 21 | (17.1%) |
| Regional enteritis +/− ileal resection | 4 | (3.3%) |
| Unkown cause (workup incomplete) | 2 | (1.6%) |

[a] Patients admitted to Harlem or Presbyterian Hospitals, 1969–1977.
[b] Includes one patient who also had Waldenstrom's macroglobulinemia with ileal improvement.
[c] Includes nine patients with combined $B_{12}$ and folate deficiency.

pairment of the pH-dependent uptake by ileal microvillus receptors, or increased association of cobalamins with R-binders at lowered intestinal pH.

When the physiology of cobalamin absorption is viewed from a clinical standpoint, it is apparent that the absolute requirements for $B_{12}$ absorption from food are the presence of intrinsic factor and an intact ileum. In the United States, virtually 100% of patients who develop clinically significant deficiency of the vitamin lack intrinsic factor, or have ileal disease or jejunal bacterial overgrowth (Table 2).

## FOLIC ACID ABSORPTION

Malabsorption of folic acid is a much less frequent cause of clinically important lack of the vitamin than is the case with cobalamins. Nonetheless, folate deficiency due to impaired absorption is likely to occur in certain patients, especially those with extensive mucosal disease of the duodenum and jejunum.

## FOLATES IN FOOD

The normal diet of industrialized countries contains about 200 $\mu$g of total folate (57, 58). In almost all of the dietary folate, the double bonds on the pyrazine ring of the pteridine moiety of folic acid are reduced, and a methyl or formyl group is attached at the $N_5$ or $N_{10}$ position (59–61). In most foods that have been well characterized, such as lettuce, cabbage, liver, or orange juice, most of the folate is present as polyglutamates with five or more glutamate residues added in gamma-carboxyl linkage to the single glutamic acid found in pteroylmonoglutamate (60). Some foods, however, such as soybeans and milk, contain mainly monoglutamate forms (60). Substantial conversion of polyglutamates to monoglutamates by endogenous hydrolases was found to occur in chicken liver during 5 days of storage at icebox temperature (62). Very little pteroylglutamic acid or other oxidized folates are present in foods (60, 61).

Prolonged boiling of foods may cause substantial losses of total folate content, primarily as a result of leaching of folate into cooking water (63). The previously reported loss of "free" (i.e., monoglutamate) folate with the cooking of some foods, such as cabbage, may have been an artifact of the experimental conditions (60, 64).

Few reliable data are available concerning the availability of folate from different items of the diet under experimental conditions resembling the real-life intake of foods. The best currently available methods require continuous high level saturation with dietary folate and the ingestion of huge amounts of the foods under study in order to obtain semireproducible values for urinary folate excretion. Under these conditions, the availability of folate from various food items has varied widely (65–67).

Folate-binding proteins are present in foods, such as the binder present in milk which is currently in use in most radioassays for serum folate, but little is known about whether these binders enhance or retard folate absorption. Other dietary items, such as cellulose, may conceivably adsorb dietary folates and impair their assimilation (68).

## HYDROLYSIS OF POLYGLUTAMATE FOLATES

With the recent development of biochemical techniques for the solid- or liquid-phase synthesis of radiolabeled polyglutamates, important information has been generated about the mechanism of absorption of folates in humans (69, 70). Purified polyglutamates have been shown to be substantially absorbed in human subjects, although less efficiently than monoglutamates (70–72). In jejunal perfusion studies in normal subjects and patients with sprue syndromes, the luminal disappearance of polyglutamate folates was less rapid than that of equimolar amounts of monoglutamates, suggesting a limiting effect of hydrolysis on absorption (71–73). Hydrolysis of polyglutamates to monoglutamates appears to be an obligatory step in the absorption of folates from polyglutamates. Polyglutamate forms of folate, with the possible exception of folyldiglutamate, do not appear in the mesenteric circulation during absorption (74, 75).

When the human small intestine is perfused with polyglutamate folates, hydrolysis products with decreasing number of glutamate residues down to the monoglutamate form appear in the gut lumen distal to the site of perfusion. Since the intestinal fluids obtained from human subjects contain insignificant hydrolytic activity, the most reasonable interpretation is that hydrolysis occurs on or inside the intestinal cell. The rapid luminal appearance of these hydrolytic products suggests strongly that the hydrolysis goes on at the cell surface. Such an interpretation would require the presence of an active hydrolytic enzyme (called by various investigators "conjugase," "pteroyl polyglutamyl hydrolase," or "gamma-glutamyl-carboxy-peptidase") on the cell surface. Most workers, however, have reported that enzyme activity in intestinal cells is largely localized to lysosomal fractions (76, 77). This dilemma apepars to have been resolved recently by the report of Reisenauer and colleagues of two separate enzyme activities in human jejunum, one intracellular with a pH optimum of 4.5 (presumably lysosomal), and the other localized to brush border membranes, with a pH optimum of 7.5 (78).

Inhibitors of polyglutamate folate absorption have been described in yeast (possibly due to nucleic acids) (79), pulses (80), and orange juice (possibly related to changes in gut pH under experimental conditions in which massive amounts were ingested) (65, 66). The mechanism of action and clinical importance of such inhibitors remain to be defined.


## MONOGLUTAMATE ABSORPTION

Monoglutamate folates present in the diet as well as those generated by intestinal cell hydrolysis of polyglutamates appear to share a common final pathway—that of monoglutamate transport across the cell (70). Considerable conflicting evidence from many laboratories has accumulated from in vitro and in vivo studies in various species of the mechanism of monoglutamate transport (70). In man, for example, evidence for a saturable mechanism and for transport against a concentration gradient has been obtained from perfusion studies (81). On the other hand, the total amounts of folate absorbed from tritiated monoglutamates appear to be similar over a dose range of 25 to 3000 $\mu$g (82).

Experiments showing greater absorption of the natural isomer of 5-methyl-tetrahydrofolate than the unnatural isomer in human subjects have been offered in support of the concept of a carrier-mediated mechanism (83). The most convincing argument for the existence of a specific transport mechanism is the occurrence of rare cases of congenital isolated folate malabsorption in the absence of other disturbances of intestinal function (84, 85). Such patients have been shown to have markedly impaired absorption of polyglutamate and monoglutamate folates (including oxidized, reduced, methylated, and formylated forms), and require huge doses of oral folic acid to prevent recurrence of megaloblastic anemia. All four reported patients have had mental retardation, in varying degrees, and transport of folates into the central nervous system also appears to be abnormal (84).

The controversy over how monoglutamate folates are transported may be partly a reflection of differing experimental conditions (70) but may best be resolved by postulating the existence of a dual mechanism, that is, a carrier-mediated, saturable, uphill transport system for low concentrations, and passive transport at higher concentrations. There is increasing evidence for the presence of such a dual system in the rat (86, 87).

Monoglutamate folate absorption in man is depressed by alkalinization of the jejunum (88–90). It has been proposed that this is related to increased ionization of folic acid above the pK's of its glutamyl carboxyl groups, resulting in decreased passive diffusion of the nonionic form of the molecule (91), although other interpretations of the pH effect have been offered (92). The role of brush border folate-binding protein (or proteins) (93, 94) in folate absorption remains to be established. Alteration of the folic acid molecule (e.g., reduction and methylation) by the intestinal cell may occur during absorption, particularly at low concentrations, but is not obligatory for folate transport (74, 95–97).

Folates are excreted in high concentration into bile (mainly in monoglutamate forms) and are reabsorbed by the small intestine (98).

## SPRUE SYNDROMES

Folate deficiency is encountered clinically as a primary result of impaired intestinal absorption most frequently in patients with marked villous atrophy of the upper small intestine. In celiac sprue (gluten-induced enteropathy) folate malabsorption is the rule, and megaloblastic anemia is common. Depressed serum or red cell folate levels have been found to be a useful screening test for the disorder and may be a sensitive indicator of noncompliance with a gluten-free diet (99–102). In patients with celiac sprue, absorption of both polyglutamate and monoglutamate folates is impaired (72, 103–105). In jejunal perfusion studies, the rate of hydrolysis of polyglutamates was estimated to be depressed, in addition to the uptake of monoglutamates (72, 105). Many groups have found adequate or increased levels of polyglutamate hydrolase activity in whole intestinal homogenates of biopsy specimens from patients with celiac (as well as tropical) sprue (70, 104), but such assays probably reflect lysosomal enzyme levels rather than the more functionally important brush border isozyme (78). A report that the pH of the lumen of the jejunum is increased in celiac patients (106) has not been confirmed by others (99). In a subgroup of patients with celiac disease, the surface pH of jejunal biopsies (as measured in vitro) was found to be abnormally high (107). Although loss of villus cells is a likely cause of folate malabsorption in this disorder, an increase in pH at the normally acid "microclimate" of the brush border could contribute to monoglutamate malabsorption in some patients (91, 107).

Megaloblastic anemia is extremely common in patients with tropical sprue, and may be due to lack of folate, cobalamin, or both vitamins. Jejunal perfusion studies have demonstrated impaired uptake of folate from purified monoglutamates (73, 108, 109) and polyglutamates (73). The degree of abnormality of monoglutamate uptake has been variable and in some cases was demonstrable only in the presence of glucose in the perfusing solution (108, 109).

In some patients with tropical sprue in whom folate deficiency was present, absorption of crystalline monoglutamate was found to be normal (110–112). In addition, some patients who have developed deficiency on a diet rich in folates respond hematologically to tiny doses of oral folic acid (113). In addition, in some individuals with normal absorption of crystalline monoglutamate, malabsorption of a yeast polyglutamate preparation has been found (112). These observations suggest that a subgroup of patients with tropical sprue may be able to absorb purified monoglutamates but are unable to process food folates. The possible importance of conjugase inhibitors, such as pulses (80), folate-adsorbing substances (68), or folate-binding proteins in the diet of patients with the disease requires further exploration.

In another subgroup of patients with tropical sprue, isolated B$_{12}$ deficiency occurs. These patients may be protected from folic acid depletion by the production of folate by the coliform bacteria that commonly overgrow the upper small bowel in this disorder (114).


## OTHER INTESTINAL DISORDERS

In a number of other conditions in which folate deficiency may occur, folate malabsorption may be one of several factors contributing to negative vitamin balance, but not necessarily the most important one; or the contribution of malabsorption may vary from patient to patient. In regional enteritis, for example, hematologically mild to moderate folate deficiency is common (115, 116). Inadequate dietary intake may be the most important cause (115). In some patients, however, especially those with duodenal and jejunal involvement by the disease, folate malabsorption may be significant (115, 117). Therapy of the disorder with sulfasalazine, as noted below, may also impair folate assimilation (116).

Since folic acid appears to be better absorbed in humans from the upper small bowel than from the ileum, surgical resection of the duodenum and jejunum should impair folate absorption in the absence of compensatory adaptation in the ileum. That adaptation occurs for folate compounds is possible (105), but has not been established. Folate absorption has been found to be depressed in some but not all patients with jejunal resection (118–122). Deficiency of the vitamin has not been a common complication in this group of patients (perhaps a reflection of their rarity plus the use of prophylactic vitamins postoperatively). When deficiency has been encountered, other factors (such as poor dietary intake, concomitant ileal resection, or very rapid intestinal transit) may have contributed to negative folate balance (122a).

The administration of various drugs may be associated with the development of folic acid deficiency. The association of anticonvulsant therapy and folate lack is well documented, but its mechanism has not been established. Many conflicting reports of the effects of diphenylhydantoin administration on both polyglutamate and monoglutamate folate absorption have been published. An inhibitory effect of the drug on polyglutamate absorption was suggested by studies using a yeast preparation (123, 124) or a food source of folate (125) in subjects who were not presaturated with folic acid. Failure to presaturate may render such investigations invalid. In any case, these findings were not confirmed by studies in which folate absorption from synthetic polyglutamates (126, 127), orange juice (128), and yeast (in presaturated volunteers) (129) was tested. On the other hand, some workers have found that the anticonvulsant impairs monoglutamate folate absorption (88, 130–132). A claim that this impairment may be due to an elevation of small intestinal pH (88) has been denied (133). It has also been postulated, but not yet proven, that anticonvulsants may cause an alteration in folate metabolism (134).

Sulfasalazine has been shown to impair folate monoglutamate absorption by human subjects (116). The agent caused a dose-related competitive inhibition of folic acid uptake in everted rat jejunal rings (116). Whether it causes folate deficiency in patients is not yet certain, but two suggestive case reports have recently appeared (135, 136). A fall in serum

Table 3   Cause of Folate Deficiency in 194 Consecutive Cases of Megaloblastic Anemia in New York City[a]

|  | Number of Cases | |
|---|---|---|
| Alcoholism and poor diet[b] | 174 | (89.7%) |
| Poor diet | 4 | (2.1%) |
| Pregnancy (nonalcoholic) | 2 | (1.0%) |
| Tropical sprue[c] | 11 | (5.7%) |
| Unknown cause[d] | 3 | (1.5%) |

[a] Patients admitted to Harlem or Presbyterian Hospitals, 1969–1977.
[b] Includes three pregnant patients, four on anticonvulsants, one with cancer.
[c] Includes nine patients with combined $B_{12}$ and folate deficiency also listed in Table 2.
[d] Includes two patients on oral contraceptive therapy.

and red cell folate concentrations occurs in individuals taking the nonabsorbable anion exchange resin cholestyramine (137). Although an effect on folate absorption has not yet been shown experimentally, it is likely that this agent interferes with monoglutamate or polyglutamate absorption (or enterohepatic recycling) as a result of its ability to bind anions. The evidence that oral contraceptive drugs interfere with folate absorption is unconvincing (138).

In a number of other conditions associated with small bowel dysfunction, abnormal results of folic acid absorption tests have been reported in certain patients, but anemia due to folate deficiency has not been encountered clinically. These conditions include scleroderma (119), amyloidosis (119), diabetic enteropathy (119), congestive heart failure (139), Whipple's disease (119), partial gastrectomy (140), and hypoparathyroidism (119). Folate malabsorption may also occur in patients with lymphomas (119, 141) and (rarely) with the blind loop syndrome (142), but it has yet to be convincingly demonstrated that deficiency occurs as a result of malabsorption in these settings.

## ALCOHOLISM AND FOLATE DEFICIENCY

The great majority of patients who develop megaloblastic anemia due to folate deficiency in New York City are chronic alcoholics who have been drinking heavily and eating poorly (Table 3). Jejunal folate uptake, as assessed by perfusion studies, is usually abnormal at the time of admission to hospital in such patients (143), as is xylose absorption (144). Folate deficiency is more likely to be the cause than the result of folate malabsorption in this setting (144, 145). The administration of alcohol to human volunteers along with a folate-supplemented diet has been shown to have little effect on folic acid absorption (145, 146), and ethanol acts as a folate antagonist regardless of whether folate is given orally or parenterally (147).

On the other hand, when alcohol is given chronically along with a folate-poor diet, folic acid malabsorption develops, which is reversible by folic acid supplementation even though ethanol feeding is continued (145). Folate deficiency may impair folate absorption by producing a megaloblastic gut (148). The acute administration of ethanol causes an abrupt fall in serum folate concentration (149), and it has been suggested from experiments in rats that this is due to interference with folate excretion into bile by the liver, which leads to interruption of the enterohepatic circulation (150). Whether reabsorption of biliary folate is a major determinant of serum folate levels in humans is unknown.

Since folic acid added to wine was well absorbed by chronic alcoholics, the morbidity and mortality due to folate deficiency in this country could be largely eliminated by fortification of alcoholic beverages with the vitamin (151).

# REFERENCES

1. J. F. Adams, F. McEwan, and A. Wilson, *Br. J. Nutr.*, **29**, 65 (1973).

2. L. E. Ericson and Z. G. Banhidi, *Acta Chem. Scand.*, **7**, 167 (1953).

3. S. J. Baker, quoted in R. P. Britt, C. Harper, and G. H. Spray, *Quart. J. Med.*, **160**, 511 (1971).

4. J. Farquharson and J. F. Adams, *Br. J. Nutr.*, **36**, 127 (1976).

5. J. F. Adams, S. Ross, L. Mervyn, K. Boddy, and P. King, *Scand. J. Gastro.* **6**, 249 (1971).

6. R. M. Heyssel, R. C. Bozian, W. J. Darby, and M. C. Bell, *Am. J. Clin. Nutr.*, **18**, 176 (1966).

7. A. Doscherholmen, J. McMahon, and D. Ripley, *Am. J. Clin. Nutr.* **31**, 825 (1978).

8. A. Doscherholmen and W. R. Swaim, *Gastroenterology*, **64**, 913 (1973).

9. A. Doscherholmen, J. McMahon, and D. Ripley, *Proc. Soc. Exp. Biol. Med.*, **149**, 987 (1975).

10. A. Doscherholmen, J. McMahon, and D. Ripley, *Brit. J. Haemat.*, **33**, 261 (1976).

11. P. G. Reizenstein, *Acta Med. Scand.*, **165**, 481 (1959).

12. B. A. Cooper and W. B. Castle, *J. Clin. Invest.*, **39**, 199 (1960).

13. S. G. Schade and R. F. Schilling, *Am. J. Clin. Nutr.*, **20**, 636 (1967).

14. J. F. Adams, E. H. Kennedy, J. Thompson, and J. Williamson, *Br. J. Nutr.*, **22**, 111 (1968).

15. K. Mahmud, D. Ripley, and A. Doscherholmen, *J.A.M.A.*, **216**, 1167 (1971).

16. A. M. Streeter, B. Duriappah, R. Boyle, B. J. O'Neill, and M. T. Pheils, *Am. J. Surg.*, **128**, 340 (1974).

17. A. M. Streeter, H. Y. Shum, V. M. Duncombe, J. W. Hewson, and M. E. C. Thorpe, *Med. J. Aust.*, **1**, 54 (1976).

18. R. Carmel, *Ann. Intern. Med.*, **88**, 647 (1978).

19. C. King, J. Leibach, and P. Toskes, *Gastroenterology*, **72**, 1080 (1977).

20. J. F. Adams and E. J. Cartwright, *Gut*, **4**, 32 (1963).

21. J. Salokannel, *Acta Med. Scand.*, **189**, Suppl. 517 (1971).

22. R. H. Donaldson, "Mechanisms of Malabsorption of Cobalamin," in B. M. Babior, Ed., *Cobalamin*, Wiley, New York, 1975, p. 335.

23. J. D. Hines, A. V. Hoffbrand, and D. L. Mollin, *Am. J. Med.*, **43**, 555 (1967).

24. M. S. Rose and I. Chanarin, *Brit. Med. J.*, **1**, 25, (1971).

25. R. O. McIntyre, L. W. Sullivan, G. H. Jeffries, and R. H. Silver, *New Engl. J. Med.*, **272**, 98 (1965).

26. M. Katz, S. K. Lee, and B. A. Cooper, *New Engl. J. Med.*, **287**, 425 (1972).

27. R. H. Allen, *Progress in Hematology*, **9**, 57 (1975).

28. R. H. Allen, B. Seetharam, E. Podell, and D. H. Alpers, *J. Clin. Invest.*, **61**, 47 (1978).

29. W. Veeger, J. Abels, N. Hellemans, and H. D. Nieweg, *New Engl. J. Med.*, **267**, 1341 (1962).

30. P. P. Toskes, J. Hansell, J. Cerda, and J. J. Deren, *New Engl. J. Med.*, **284**, 627 (1971).

31. C. Matuchansky, J. C. Rambaud, R. Modigliani, and J. J. Bernier, *Gastroenterology*, **67**, 406 (1974).

32. P. P. Toskes, J. J. Deren, and M. E. Conrad, *J. Clin. Invest.*, **52**, 1660 (1973).

33. R. H. Allen, B. Seetharam, N. C. Allen, E. R. Podell, and D. H. Alpers, *J. Clin. Invest.*, **62**, 1628 (1978).

34. P. A. McIntyre, M. V. Sachs, J. R. Krevans, and C. L. Conley, *Arch. Intern. Med.*, **98**, 541 (1956).

35. J. T. Henderson, R. R. G. Warwick, J. D. Simpson, and D. J. C. Shearman, *Lancet*, **2**, 241 (1972).

36. C. R. Kapadia, P. Bhat, E. Jacob, and S. J. Baker, *Gut*, **16**, 988 (1975).

37. R. A. Giannella, S. A. Broitman, and N. Zamcheck, *J. Clin. Invest.*, **50**, 1100 (1971).

38. R. A. Giannella, S. A. Broitman, and N. Zamcheck, *Gastroenterology*, **62**, 255 (1972).

39. L. J. Brandt, L. H. Bernstein, and A. Wagle, *Ann. Intern. Med.*, **87**, 546 (1977).

40. J. Lindenbaum, *Gastroenterology*, **64**, 637 (1973).

40a. V. Herbert, *J. Clin. Invest.*, **38**, 102 (1959).

40b. S. P. Rothenberg, *J. Clin. Invest.*, **47**, 913 (1968).

41. M. Katz and B. A. Cooper, *J. Clin. Invest.*, **54**, 733 (1974).

41a. R. Cotter, S. P. Rothenberg, and J. P. Weiss, *Biochim. Biophys. Acta*, **490**, 19 (1977).

120     Gastrointestinal Diseases that Affect Nutrition

41b. G. Marcoullis and R. Grasbeck, *Biochim. Biophys. Acta,* **499,** 309 (1977).

41c. S. Yamada, H. Itaya, O. Nakagawa, and M. Fakuda, *Biochim. Biophys. Acta,* **496,** 571 (1977).

42. C. H. Hagedorn and D. H. Alpers, *Gastroenterology,* **73,** 1019 (1977).

42a. S. P. Rothenberg, H. Weisberg, and A. Fiarra, *J. Lab. Clin. Med.,* **79,** 587 (1972).

42b. C. R. Kapadia and R. M. Donaldson, *Gastroenterology,* **76,** 1163 (1979).

43. T. J. Peters and A. V. Hoffbrand, *Brit. J. Haemat.,* **19,** 369 (1970).

44. I. Chanarin, M. Muir, A. Hughes, and A. V. Hoffbrand, *Brit. Med. J.,* **1,** 1453 (1978).

44a. S. P. Rothenberg, J. P. Weiss, and R. Cotter, *Brit. J. Haemat.,* **40,** 401 (1978).

44b. M. Katz and R. O'Brien, *J. Lab. Clin. Med.,* **94,** 817 (1979).

45. N. Hakami, P. E. Neiman, G. P. Canellos, and J. Lazerson, *New Engl. J. Med.,* **285,** 1163 (1971).

46. W. H. Hitzig, U. Dohmann, H. J. Pluss, and D. Vischer, *J. Ped.,* **85,** 622 (1974)

47. J. F. Burman, D. L. Mollin, R. A. Sladden, N. Sourial, and M. Greany, *Brit. J. Haemat.,* **35,** 676 (1977).

48. I. L. Mackenzie, R. M. Donaldson, Jr., J. S. Trier, and V. I. Mathan, *New Engl. J. Med.,* **286,** 1021 (1972).

49. P. Foroozan and J. S. Trier, *New Engl. J. Med.,* **277,** 553 (1967).

50. J. Lindenbaum, J. F. Pezzimenti, and N. Shea, *Ann. Intern. Med.,* **80,** 326 (1974).

51. P. P. Toskes and J. J. Deren, *Gastroenterology,* **62,** 1232 (1972).

52. E. D. Jacobson, R. B. Chodos, and W. W. Faloon, *Am. J. Med.* **28,** 524 (1960).

53. D. I. Webb, R. B. Chodos, C. Q. Mahar, and W. W. Faloon, *New Engl. J. Med.,* **279,** 845 (1968).

54. G. H. Tomkin, *Brit. Med. J.,* **3,** 673 (1973).

55. J. Lindenbaum and C. S. Lieber, *Nature,* **224,** 806 (1969).

56. S. Schimoda, D. R. Saunders, and C. E. Rubin, *Gastroenterology,* **55,** 705 (1968).

57. K. Hoppner, B. Lampi, and D. C. Smith, in Workshop on Human Folate Requirements, *Folic Acid,* National Academy of Sciences, Washington, D.C., 1977, pp. 69–81.

58. V. Herbert, in Workshop on Human Folate Requirements, *Folic Acid,* National Academy of Sciences, Washington, D.C., 1977, p. 286.

59. C. E. Butterworth, Jr., R. Santini, Jr., and W. B. Frommeyer, Jr., *J. Clin. Invest.,* **42,** 1929 (1963).

60. E. L. R. Stokstad, Y. S. Shin, and T. Tamura, in Workshop on Human Folate Requirements, *Folic Acid,* National Academy of Sciences, Washington, D.C., 1977, p. 56.

61. J. Perry, *Brit. J. Haemat.,* **28,** 435 (1971).

62. B. Reed, D. Weir, and J. Scott, *Am. J. Clin. Nutr.,* **29,** 1393 (1976).

63. Y. J. Huskisson and F. P. Retief, *S. Afr. Med. J.,* **44,** 362 (1970).

64. J. D. Malin, *Proc. Nutr. Soc.,* **35,** 143A (1976).

65. T. Tamura and E. L. R. Stokstad, *Brit. J. Haemat.,* **25,** 513 (1973).

66 T. Tamura, Y. S. Shin, K. U. Buehring, and E. L. R. Stokstad, *Brit. J. Haemat.,* **32,** 123 (1976).

67. S. Babu and S. G. Srikantia, *Am. J. Clin. Nutr.*, **29**, 376 (1976).
68. L. Luther, R. Santini, C. Brewster, E. Perez-Santiago, and C. E. Butterworth, Jr., *Alabama J. Med. Sci.*, **2**, 389 (1965).
69. C. E. Butterworth, Jr., C. M. Baugh, and C. Krumdieck, *J. Clin. Invest.*, **48**, 1131 (1969).
70. I. H. Rosenberg, *Clinics in Haemat.*, **5**, 589 (1976).
71. C. H. Halsted, C. M. Baugh, and C. E. Butterworth, Jr., *Gastroenterology*, **68**, 261 (1975).
72. C. H. Halsted, A. M. Reisenauer, J. J. Romero, D. S. Cantor, and B. Ruebner, *J. Clin. Invest.*, **59**, 933 (1977).
73. J. J. Corcino, A. M. Reisenauer, and C. H. Halsted, *J. Clin. Invest.*, **58**, 298 (1976).
74. C. M. Baugh, C. L. Krumdieck, H. J. Baker, and C. E. Butterworth, Jr., *J. Clin. Invest.*, **50**, 2009 (1971).
75. M. Jägerstad, H. Dencker, and A. K. Westesson, *Scand. J. Gastro.*, **11**, 283 (1976).
76. A. V. Hoffbrand and T. J. Peters, *Biochim. Biophys. Acta*, **192**, 479 (1969).
77. I. H. Rosenberg and H. A. Godwin, *Gastroenterology*, **60**, 445 (1971).
78. A. M. Reisenauer, C. L. Krumdieck, and C. H. Halsted, *Science*, **198**, 196 (1977).
79. I. H. Rosenberg and H. A. Godwin, *J. Clin. Invest.*, **50**, 78a (1971).
80. C. E. Butterworth, Jr., A. J. Newman, and C. L. Krumdieck, *Trans. Amer. Clin. Climatol. Assoc.*, **86**, 11 (1974).
81. G. W. Hepner, C. C. Booth, J. Cowan, A. V. Hoffbrand, and D. L. Mollin, *Lancet*, **2**, 302 (1968).
82. I. Chanarin, *The Megaloblastic Anaemias*, Blackwell, Philadelphia, 1969, p. 849.
83. D. G. Weir, J. P. Brown, D. S. Freedman, and J. M. Scott, *Clin. Sci. Molecular Med.*, **45**, 625 (1973).
84. P. Lanzkowsky, *Am. J. Med.*, **580**, (1970).
85. P. J. Santiago-Borrero, R. Santini, Jr., E. Perez-Santiago, and N. Maldonado, *J. Ped.*, **82**, 450 (1973).
86. C. H. Halsted, K. Bhanthumnavin, and E. Mezey, *J. Nutr.*, **104**, 1674 (1974).
87. G. Jeelani Dhar, J. Selhub, C. Gay, and I. Rosenberg, *Gastroenterology*, **72**, A-26/1049 (1977).
88. A. Benn, C. H. J. Swan, W. T. Cooke, J. A. Blair, A. J. Matty, and M. E. Smith, *Brit. Med. J.*, **1**, 148 (1971).
89. J. F. Mackenzie and R. I. Russell, *Clin. Sci. Molecular Med.*, **51**, 363 (1976).
90. S. Dutta and R. M. Russell, *Gastroenterology*, **70**, A-122/980 (1976).
91. J. A. Blair and A. J. Matty, *Clinics in Gastroenterology*, **3**, 183 (1974).
92. I. H. Rosenberg, *Abstr. Sixth Internat. Symp. Chem. Biol. Pteridines*, La Jolla, 1978.
93. G. I. Leslie and P. B. Rowe, *Biochemistry*, **11**, 1696 (1972).
94. B. C. Das and S. A. Shaw, *Gastroenterology*, **72**, A-20/1043 (1977).
95. V. M. Whitehead and B. A. Cooper, *Brit. J. Haemat.*, **13**, 679 (1967).
96. V. M. Whitehead, R. Pratt, A. Viallet, and B. A. Cooper, *Brit. J. Haemat.*, **22**, 63 (1972).
97. R. J. Leeming, H. Portman-Graham, and J. A. Blair, *J. Clin. Path.*, **25**, 491 (1972).

98. R. F. Pratt and B. A. Cooper, *J. Clin. Invest.*, **50**, 455 (1971).

99. P. E. Mortimer, J. S. Stewart, A. P. Norman, and C. C. Booth, *Brit. Med. J.*, **3**, 7 (1968).

100. A. S. McNeish and M. L. N. Willoughby, *Lancet*, **1**, 442, (1969).

101. D. G. Weir and D. O'B. Hourihane, *Gut*, **15**, 450 (1974).

102. A. V. Hoffbrand, *Clinics in Gastroenterology*, **3**, 71 (1974).

103. I. H. Rosenberg, H. A. Godwin, R. M. Russell, and J. L. Franklin, *J. Clin. Invest.*, **53**, 66a (1974).

104. A. V. Hoffbrand, A. P. Douglas, L. Fry, and J. S. Stewart, *Brit. Med. J.*, **4**, 85 (1970).

105. C. H. Halsted, A. M. Reisenauer, B. Shane, and T. Tamura, *Gut*, **19**, 886 (1978).

106. A. Benn and W. T. Cooke, *Scand. J. Gastro.*, **6**, 313 (1971).

107. M. L. Lucas, B. T. Cooper, F. H. Lei, I. T. Johnson, G. K. T. Holmes, J. A. Blair, and W. T. Cooke, *Gut*, **19**, 735 (1978).

108. C. D. Gerson, N. Cohen, N. Brown, J. Lindenbaum, G. W. Hepner, and H. D. Janowitz, *Am. J. Dig. Dis.*, **19**, 911 (1974).

109. J. J. Corcino, G. Coll, and F. A. Klipstein, *Blood*, **45**, 577 (1975).

110. D. E. Paterson, R. David, and S. J. Baker, *Brit. J. Radiol.*, **38**, 181 (1965).

111. F. A. Klipstein, *Blood*, **34**, 191 (1969).

112. A. V. Hoffbrand, T. F. Necheles, N. Maldonado, E. Horta, and R. Santini, *Brit. Med. J.*, **2**, 543 (1969).

113. T. W. Sheehy, M. E. Rubini, E. Perez-Santiago, R. Santini, Jr., and J. Haddock, *Blood*, **18**, 623 (1961).

114. F. A. Klipstein and I. M. Samloff, *Am. J. Clin. Nutr.*, **19**, 237 (1966).

115. A. V. Hoffbrand, J. S. Stewart, C. C. Booth, and D. L. Mollin, *Brit. Med. J.*, **2**, 71 (1968).

116. J. L. Franklin and I. H. Rosenberg, *Gastroenterology*, **64**, 517 (1973).

117. E. V. Cox, M. J. Meynell, W. T. Cooke, and R. Gaddie, *Gastroenterology*, **35**, 390 (1958).

118. C. C. Booth, *Postgrad. Med. J.*, **37**, 725 (1961).

119. F. A. Klipstein, *Bull. N.Y. Acad. Med.*, **42**, 638 (1966).

120. H. Baker, A. D. Thomson, S. Feingold, and O. Frank, *Am. J. Clin. Nutr.*, **22**, 124 (1969).

121. D. Pavesio, *Minerva Pediat.*, **17**, 1488 (1965).

122. L. Elsborg and P. Bastrup-Madsen, *Scand. J. Gastroent.*, **11**, 333 (1976).

122a. A. V. Hoffbrand, *J. Clin. Path.*, **24**, Suppl. 5, 66 (1971).

123. A. V. Hoffbrand and T. F. Necheles, *Lancet*, **2**, 528 (1968).

124. I. H. Rosenberg, H. A. Godwin, R. R. Streiff, and W. B. Castle, *Lancet*, **2**, 530 (1968)

125. P. Reizenstein and L. Lund, *Scand. J. Haemat.*, **11**, 158 (1973).

126. C. Fehling, M. Jagerstad, K. Lindstrand, and A. K. Westesson, *Clin. Sci.*, **44**, 595 (1973).

127. C. M. Houlihan, J. M. Scott, P. H. Boyle, and D. G. Weir, *Gut*, **13**, 189 (1972).

128. E. W. Nelson, J. J. Cerda, B. J. Wilder, and R. R. Streiff, *Am. J. Clin. Nutr.*, **31**, 82 (1978).

129. J. Perry and I. Chanarin, *Gut,* **13,** 544 (1972).

130. M. B. Dahlke and E. Mertens-Roessler, *Blood,* **30,** 341 (1967).

131. C. D. Gerson, G. W. Hepner, N. Brown, N. Cohen, V. Herbert, and H. D. Janowitz, *Gastroenterology,* **63,** 246 (1972).

132. L. Elsborg, *Acta. Haemat.,* **52,** 2 (1974).

133. W. F. Doe, A. V. Hoffbrand, P. I. Reid, and J. M. Scott, *Brit. Med. J.,* **1,** 669 (1971).

134. D. Labadarios, J. W. T. Dickerson, D. V. Parke, E. G. Lucas, and G. H. Obuwa, *Brit. J. Clin. Pharmac.,* **5,** 167 (1978).

135. R. E. Schneider and L. Beeley, *Brit. Med. J.,* **2,** 1638 (1977).

136. S. P. Kane and M. A. Boots, *Brit. Med. J.,* **4,** 1287 (1977).

137. R. J. West and J. K. Lloyd, *Gut,* **16,** 93 (1975).

138. J. Lindenbaum, N. Whitehead, and F. Reyner, *Am. J. Clin. Nutr.,* **28,** 346 (1975).

139. R. D. Hyde and C. A. E. H. Loehry, *Gut,* **9,** 717 (1968).

140. L. Elsborg, *Scand. J. Gastroent.,* **9,** 271 (1974).

141. W. R. Pitney, R. A. Joske, and W. L. MacKinnon, *J. Clin. Path.,* **13,** 440 (1960).

142. C. R. Barrett, Jr. and P. R. Holt, *Am. J. Med.,* **41,** 629 (1966).

143. C. H. Halsted, E. A. Robles, and E. Mezey, *New Engl. J. Med.,* **285,** 701 (1971).

144. E. Baraona and J. Lindenbaum, in C. S. Lieber, Ed., *Metabolic Aspects of Alcoholism,* MTP Press, Lancaster, Pa., 1977, p. 81

145. C. H. Halsted, E. A. Robles, and E. Mezey, *Gastroenterology,* **64,** 526 (1973).

146. J. Lindenbaum, in C. S. Lieber, Ed., *Metabolic Aspects of Alcoholism,* MTP Press, Lancaster, Pa., 1977, p. 215.

147. L. W. Sullivan and V. Herbert, *J. Clin. Invest.,* **43,** 2048 (1964).

148. J. A. Hermos, W. H. Adams, Y. K. Liu, L. W. Sullivan, and J. S. Trier, *Ann. Intern. Med.* **76,** 957 (1972).

149. E. R. Eichner and R. S. Hillman, *J. Clin. Invest.,* **52,** 584 (1973).

150. R. S. Hillman, R. McGriffin, and C. Campbell, *Trans. Assn. Amer. Phys.,* **90,** 145 (1977).

151. J. D. Kaunitz and J. Lindenbaum, *Ann. Intern. Med.,* **87,** 542 (1977).

# 8

# Malnutrition and Inflammatory Bowel Disease

RICHARD J. GRAND, M.D.

Harvard Medical School and The Children's Hospital Medical Center, Boston, Massachusetts.

The chronic inflammatory bowel diseases, ulcerative colitis and Crohn's disease, are being recognized with increasing frequency. It is still not clear whether this is a true increase in worldwide incidence of these diseases (as suggested by data from some countries) (1, 2) or a reflection of increased awareness on the part of physicians and other health care workers. Indeed, it is also not clear whether these disorders are two separate entities or merely parts of the spectrum of one disease (3). Even after extensive studies, a definitive diagnosis is often difficult to establish, and may be based on arbitrary criteria. For both conditions, the etiology is unknown.

Many clinical features are common to both disorders, especially diarrhea, gastrointestinal blood and protein loss, abdominal pain, weight loss, fever, anemia, and growth failure in children when disease is severe. In addition, both types of inflammatory bowel disease have a familial distribution, and both are associated with a certain number of extraintestinal manifestations, involving particularly the eyes, joints, skin, and liver.

Supported in part by a Clinical Research Center Grant (#PR-00128) from the National Institutes of Health, by a grant from the National Foundation for Ileitis and Colitis, and gifts from the Hazel Dell Foundation, Inc., and the Daughters of Penelope (District 8).

**Table 1    Causes of Malnutrition in Inflammatory Bowel Disease**

1. Inadequate intake
    Anorexia
    Altered taste
    Increased pain
    Increased diarrhea
2. Excessive losses
    Protein losing enteropathy
    Gastrointestinal bleeding
    Steatorrhea
3. Malabsorption
    Protein
    Carbohydrate
    Fat
    Bacterial overgrowth
    Minerals
    Vitamins
4. Increased requirements
    Fever
    Fistulae
    Repletion of stores
    Growth

Ulcerative colitis and Crohn's disease demonstrate a bimodal distribution in age at onset, the peaks occurring between 10 and 30 years of age, and again between 50 and 60 years of age. Details of classification and definition of these disorders have been published recently by Schachter and Kirsner (3). Ulcerative colitis, by definition, is limited to the colon, with minimal if any involvement of the terminal ileum. By contrast, Crohn's disease can occur in any portion of the gastrointestinal tract; approximately 35% of patients have disease in the small bowel alone, 5% have disease in the colon alone, and 60% have involvement of both small bowel and colon. Careful clinical studies have pointed out that malnutrition and intestinal malabsorption tend to be more common in patients whose Crohn's disease involves proximal segments of small intestine (4).

## ETIOLOGY OF MALNUTRITION IN INFLAMMATORY BOWEL DISEASE

Malnutrition in patients with inflammatory bowel disease is a multifactorial problem, and it is often impossible to identify a single cause in

**Table 2    Malabsorption in Crohn's Disease**[a]

|  | Adults | Children |
|---|---|---|
| **1. Protein** | | |
| Protein loss | 21/30 (70%) | 12/17 (70%) |
| Serum albumin <3.3% | 43/83 (52%) | 9/17 (52%) |
| **2. Carbohydrate** | | |
| Xylose | 31/80 (40%) | 3/18 (16%) |
| Lactose | 2/23 (10%) | 3/17 (17%) |
| **3. Bacterial overgrowth** | 11/36 (30%) | |
| **4. Fat** | | |
| Serum carotene ↓ | 44/47 (94%) | |
| Fecal fat | 34/79 (43%) | 5/17 (29%) |
| **5. Vitamins and minerals** | | |
| Folic acid (serum, decreased) | 64/83 (77%) | 6/10 (60%) |
| Vitamin $B_{12}$ (abnormal Schilling) | 40/69 (58%) | 6/11 |55%) |
| Serum iron decreased | 15/26 (58%) | 7/10 (70%) |
| Serum calcium decreased | 11/63 (17%) | 2/11 (18%) |
| Negative calcium balance | 4/31 (13%) | 2/11 (18%) |

[a] References (4–9, 14).

individual cases. The major factors involved are listed in Table 1 and include inadequate intake, excessive losses, malabsorption, and increased nutritional requirements (4–9).

Inadequate intake may occur in patients with inflammatory bowel disease because of anorexia induced by chronic illness or the presence of chronic inflammation. Often patients may be unwilling to eat because of increases in diarrhea accompanying the ingestion of food, or because of exacerbation of abdominal pain following meals.

Excessive losses of blood and protein in the stool and increased fecal losses of cellular constituents result from chronic inflammation and ulceration of the intestinal mucosa. Increased fecal excretion of dietary constituents may also occur in the presence of malabsorption.

In addition to these factors, certain aspects of therapy for Crohn's disease may contribute to nitrogen losses. For example, large doses of corticosteroids are often used to control inflammatory disease. Ample evidence demonstrates that increased excretion of nitrogen and loss of protein from the carcass of experimental animals can occur after administration of pharmacologic doses of corticosteroids (10). Nevertheless, it has been observed repeatedly that many patients with inflammatory bowel disease demonstrate marked improvement in nutritional status during courses of therapy with corticosteroids (11–13). The controlling factor in such patients may actually be caloric or nitrogen intake, but the relative contribution of each of these in overcoming the effects of corticosteroids or in the repletion of body stores has not been intensively studied.

Defects in intestinal absorption are common in patients with Crohn's disease, but less common in patients with ulcerative colitis. Particularly in Crohn's disease, there is a striking correlation between the location of disease and the degree of malabsorption. Those patients with small bowel disease tend to have more malabsorption than those with disease elsewhere in the intestine. The most marked abnormalities are found in patients with jejunal involvement.

The prevalence and characteristics of malabsorption in patients with Crohn's disease are shown in Table 2. Gastrointestinal protein loss, as reflected by abnormal fecal excretion of $^{51}$chromium-labeled albumin, is extremely common, occurring in approximately 70% of children and adults with Crohn's disease. Similarly, hypoalbuminemia occurs in at least 50% of patients with Crohn's disease. Loss of blood in the stools, sloughing of damaged intestinal cells, and the exudative response to intestinal inflammation intensify the nitrogen losses.

Carbohydrate malabsorption is less common. Approximately 16% of children and 40% of adults with Crohn's disease exhibit abnormal xylose absorption tests. This reflects either mucosal injury or bacterial overgrowth, each of which must be confirmed by additional testing. Lactose absorption is abnormal in not more than 20% of patients with inflammatory bowel disease, probably reflecting the prevalence of lactose intolerance in the normal mixed white population (15). Thus, little specificity can be applied to the abnormality of this test in patients with Crohn's disease, although its presence signifies a need for investigation of mucosal function and bacterial overgrowth. Bacterial overgrowth itself occurs in approximately 30% of patients with Crohn's disease.

In regard to fat malabsorption, serum carotene levels are often low in adults with inflammatory bowel disease. This may be due to voluntary restriction of vegetables and other nutrients containing carotene pigments, or it may reflect the presence of steatorrhea. Excessive loss of fat in the stools occurs in approximately 40% of adults and 30% of children with Crohn's disease. These abnormalities are due to varying combinations of mucosal injury, bacterial overgrowth, and intraluminal bile salt deficiencies, with reduction of the bile salt pool as a consequence of ileal disease.

Reductions in serum folic acid and iron levels are common, as are aberrations in vitamin $B_{12}$ absorption signified by low Schilling test results. Hypocalcemia and negative calcium balance are usually a consequence of steatorrhea. Vitamin D absorption may also be impaired in the presence of steatorrhea. Abnormalities in zinc metabolism have been proposed as potential etiologic factors in growth failure in Crohn's disease and possibly also in the anorexia and reduced food intake (16), but no definitive data are available at present. A small number of patients with Crohn's disease and growth failure have had reduced serum zinc levels, but many patients studied by us with the same clinical findings have had normal serum zinc levels (14). As for other heavy metals, marked magnesium losses often complicate active inflammatory bowel disease (17, 18), and the abnormality should be searched for in all patients with inflammatory bowel disease.

Increased nutritional requirements may be present as a response to fever, increased inflammatory activity, intestinal fistulae, or (in children) the added stress of growth. Indeed, abnormalities in growth represent the major manifestation of chronic malnutrition in pediatric patients with inflammatory bowel disease.

## MALNUTRITION AND GROWTH FAILURE IN CHILDREN WITH INFLAMMATORY BOWEL DISEASE

Severe impairment of linear growth, lack of weight gain, retarded bone development, and delayed onset of sexual maturation are seen in 15–30% of patients under the age of 21 years with Crohn's disease and a smaller number with ulcerative colitis (19). It is not uncommon to find growth failure preceding clinical evidence of bowel diseases often by years. In the series of McCaffery and colleagues of 130 patients with inflammatory bowel disease under 21 years of age, 22 patients had growth failure so severe as to place them more than two standard deviations below the mean height for age. Nineteen of these patients had Crohn's disease; three had ulcerative colitis (20). In our own clinic, we have had the opportunity to study 37 children and adolescents with Crohn's disease (12). These patients were selected from 140 patients with inflammatory bowel disease followed over a 15 year period. The ages of the patients at the time of diagnosis were 8 to 18 years. Of the 37 patients, 28 had Crohn's disease involving both colon and terminal ileum, 9 had disease limited to the small intestine or the stomach. When first seen, 16 of the 37 patients were at or below the 3rd percentile for weight, and only 16 of the 37 patients had reached puberty. All of the latter group were older than 14.5 years of age. Fourteen of the 37 patients had severe impairment of

**Table 3  Nutritional Classification of Growth Failure in Crohn's Disease**[a]

| % Expected weight for height | >95 | 95–87.5 | 87.5–80 | <80 |
|---|---|---|---|---|
| >90 | 3 | 4 | 3 | 1 |
| 90–80 | 2 | 1 | | 1 |
| 80–70 | | 1 | 1 | |
| <70 | | 1 | | |

[a] Data shown are the numbers of patients in each category. Calculations as suggested by Waterlow and co-workers.

linear growth; height was at or below the 3rd percentile, or linear growth had been absent for more than 1 year. Eleven of these patients were prepubertal and three were pubertal. These 14 patients represented approximately 25% of our population with Crohn's disease (approximately 65 patients at the time of study).

The nutritional classification (21) of some of these patients with growth failure and Crohn's disease is shown in Table 3. The data show that patients with Crohn's disease who fail to grow prior to puberty are indeed "nutritional dwarfs," fitting the criteria of Waterlow and co-workers (21) for chronic malnutrition. The majority of the patients, although short for age, are not markedly abnormal for weight, all but three being greater than 80% of expected weight for height. This "normal" body composition at an abnormal height appears to be a compensatory effort to conserve energy at the expense of growth. Whereas patients with chronic malnutrition have reduced somatomedin levels which rise when nutritional therapy is instituted (22), three patients with Crohn's disease studied by us had normal somatomedin levels. Thus, growth failure in inflammatory bowel disease undoubtedly has a nutritional basis but the many other factors that control growth in such patients have not been identified.

## GOALS OF NUTRITIONAL THERAPY IN INFLAMMATORY BOWEL DISEASE

Based on information presented above, one can provide the following guidelines for nutritional therapy in inflammatory bowel diseases. The major aim is to maintain metabolic homeostasis. This involves replace-

Table 4    Therapy of Malnutrition in Inflammatory Bowel Disease

---

1. Food
2. Oral supplements
3. Nasogastric infusions
4. Gastrostomy
5. Parenteral alimentation
    Peripheral
    Central

---

ment of losses, correction of deficits, and provision of sufficient nutrients to promote energy and nitrogen balance. In children, one of the major aims in this respect is to provide adequate energy, protein, and other substrates to restore normal growth or to permit catch-up growth to occur (23, 24).

## TECHNIQUES OF THERAPY OF MALNUTRITION IN INFLAMMATORY BOWEL DISEASE

The available methods of treatment of malnutrition in inflammatory bowel disease are somewhat limited. These are listed in Table 4.

The easiest way of providing nutritional supplementation is to increase the dietary intake using standard nutrients. Attractively preparing and serving food, and avoiding intensely restricted diets, will often result in increased nutritional intake. It would seem preferable for a patient with inflammatory bowel disease to eat a nutritious diet than to be overly concerned about the potential hazards of various foods whose deleterious effects have never been proven. There is no evidence that eating or avoiding specific foods influences the severity of disease or the frequency of relapses or in any way induces a remission. Therefore, in children and adolescents, it is preferable to allow the intake of hamburgers, hotdogs, french fries, and favorite beverages and achieve a normal caloric intake for age than to force a limited intake. Above all, an attempt should be made to provide a nutritious diet, containing the usual balance of nutrients, and to recommend a reasonable quantity of fiber, avoiding food fads in any form. Even when malabsorption is present, a nutritious diet can be achieved by reducing or eliminating those constituents which are poorly absorbed. However, since it is impossible to reduce the amount of meat fat consumed without also reducing dietary

**Table 5  Commercial Formulas for Oral Supplementation**[a]

| Product Manufacturer | Nutritional Content | | | | | Nutrient Sources | | |
|---|---|---|---|---|---|---|---|---|
| | Calories | Protein (g) | Fat (g) | Carbohydrate (g) | Osmolality | Protein | Fat | Carbohydrate |
| Instant Breakfast (Carnation Company) | 120 (made with whole milk) | 6.8 | 3.6 | 15.3 | <2000 | Nonfat dry milk | Whole milk | Sucrose, corn syrup solids, lactose |
| Isocal (Mead Johnson) | 100 | 3.4 | 4.4 | 13.2 | 350 | Casein, soy isolate | Soy oil 80%, medium-chain triglyceride 20% | Corn syrup solids |
| Ensure (Ross) | 100 | 3.7 | 3.7 | 14.5 | 460 | Casein, soy isolate | Corn oil | Corn syrup solids, sucrose |
| Portagen (Mead Johnson) | 100 | 3.5 | 4.8 | 11.5 | 236 | Casein | Medium-chain triglyceride 80%, corn oil | Corn syrup solids, sucrose (lactose) |
| Pregestimil (Mead Johnson) | 100 | 3.3 | 4.2 | 13 | 496 (.6 cal/cc) | Hydrolyzed casein | Medium-chain triglyceride 85.5%, corn oil 11.8%, lecithin 2.4% | Dextrose, corn syrup solids, tapioca starch |
| Vivonex HN (Eaton) | 100 | 4.2 | 0.1 | 21 | 844 (.6 cal/cc) | Crystalline amino acids | Safflower oil | Glucose oligosaccharides |
| Vivonex Standard (Eaton) | 100 | 2.0 | 0.2 | 22.6 | 500 | Crystalline amino acids | Safflower oil | Glucose, glucose oligosaccharides |
| Precision LR (Doyle) | 100 | 2.3 | 0.1 | 24.0 | 600 | Egg albumin | Soybean oil | Maltodextrin, sucrose |

[a] Prepared by Theresa Glanville, R.D., Nutrition Services, Children's Hospital Medical Center, Boston, Mass.

protein, fat-restricted diets must be constructed judiciously. In addition, according to the patient's clinical manifestations, it may be appropriate to recommend a daily multivitamin preparation, oral iron therapy, and folic acid. Patients who have had ileal resection may require parenteral administration of vitamin $B_{12}$.

When the patient is unable to increase caloric intake using food, it is appropriate to attempt oral supplementation with a commercially available liquid formula. Numerous preparations are available (with varying constituents) and it is not difficult to find one that contains the requirements of the individual patient. Table 5 lists some of these formulas. Successful supplementation of dietary intake may be achieved with such formulas; however, many patients will experience satiety when taking formulas and hence will not be able to increase significantly their total caloric intake. The more supplements they drink, the less food they eat. Under such circumstances, it will be necessary to provide caloric supplementation in a manner that does not depend on voluntary ingestion. As shown in Table 4 this may be done by nasogastric infusions, gastrostomy feedings, or parenteral alimentation either peripherally or centrally.

Nasogastric infusions used either continuously or intermittently (often at night) have been extremely effective in reversing metabolic imbalances in patients with inflammatory bowel disease. Two techniques can be used. The patient may have continual placement of a silicone rubber tube of small diameter which can be taped to the cheek and used as needed. Alternatively, the patient can learn to pass such a catheter in the evening and be taught to infuse a liquid formula overnight, removing the tube in the morning on awakening. This technique has been very helpful in the management of children with glycogen storage disease who infuse only high concentrations of glucose (25), but the technique can be applied to the administration of a more balanced nutrient source. If the patient does not tolerate this form of therapy, and if the patient is considered a good operative risk, a gastrostomy can be placed for either continuous or intermittent liquid formula or blenderized tube feedings. The advantage of the gastrostomy is that it is cosmetically acceptable, is easily cared for, and large increases in rate of administration of nutrients can be achieved without relying on appetite.

Often, however, patients with inflammatory bowel disease (particularly those with Crohn's disease) are unable to tolerate large quantities of alimentary supplementation because of active inflammatory disease and diarrhea. Such patients have been shown to benefit considerably from parenteral alimentation (26–28). Recent enthusiasm for peripheral alimentation with 10% glucose solutions containing 2.0–2.5% amino acids, vitamins, and minerals has suggested that this may be an acceptable form of therapy. When it is used, it may be accompanied by an intravenous lipid preparation to increase calories and supply essential fatty acids.

Alternatively, central venous alimentation (total parenteral nutrition) can be used either with or without oral feedings. We and others have clearly demonstrated that total parenteral nutrition is of value in improving the nutritional status of patients with inflammatory bowel disease as demonstrated by weight gain and improved postoperative recovery (26–28). Interestingly, these beneficial effects have occurred whether or not there was amelioration of clinical symptoms. In our experience and that of others, the greatest successes of total parenteral nutrition in facilitating control of disease occurs in those patients who have newly diagnosed Crohn's disease or who have had abdominal pain, anorexia, weight loss, and diarrhea without rectal bleeding. Indeed, total parenteral nutrition may provide remission of disease without the use of sulfasalazine or corticosteroids. By contrast, attempts to use total parenteral nutrition to achieve bowel rest in patients with frank rectal bleeding (due to ulcerative colitis or Crohn's disease) have been less successful. Although an occasional patient with active bleeding will achieve remission with a combination of sulfasalazine, corticosteroids, and total parenteral nutrition, the success rate is less frequent in this setting.

## TOTAL PARENTERAL NUTRITION AND THE TREATMENT OF GROWTH FAILURE

In addition to the indications for total parenteral nutrition in inflammatory bowel disease discussed above, we have become interested in the potential role of this mode of therapy in reversing growth failure in patients with Crohn's disease. Our interest was stimulated by the frequency of growth failure in Crohn's disease (15 to 30% of children with this diagnosis), by the fact that growth retardation may precede clinical symptoms often by years, and by reports that growth failure may occur in the absence of demonstrable malabsorption, intestinal protein loss, or endocrine dysfunction (12, 19, 20, 29). The potential effects of steroids on growth are difficult to assess in individual patients, and our previous data demonstrated that the growth after surgery for Crohn's disease was disappointing (12). In addition, it has been shown by others that administration of human growth hormone to patients with Crohn's disease and growth failure has no effect on linear growth (30).

Accordingly, we were interested in the metabolic consequences of nu-

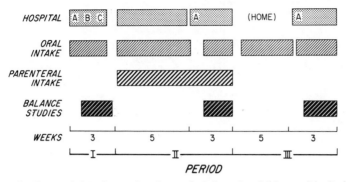

**Figure 1.** Protocol for the study of growth failure in children with Crohn's disease. Studies A: Complete blood count; serum total protein, albumin, carotene folic acid, and vitamin $B_{12}$ levels; $^{40}K$ counting; basal metabolic rate; creatinine excretion. B: Fecal fat excretion, Schilling test, xylose absorption test, $^{51}$chromium-labeled albumin. C: Thyroid and adrenal hormone levels, glucose tolerance test with insulin levels, propranolol, and glucagon challenge.

tritional therapy for growth failure and have explored changes in body composition induced by this mode of therapy. We have investigated seven patients with Crohn's disease and growth failure according to the plan of study shown in Figure 1. The letters refer to groups of laboratory investigations obtained during each period (see legend). Throughout the entire evaluation, the patients ate a self-chosen, constant, normally balanced diet containing approximately 51% carbohydrate, 35% fat, and 14% protein. Period I consisted of initial metabolic and endocrine studies with patients on an oral diet only. During Period II, patients received a total of 6 to 8 weeks of central venous hyperalimentation plus oral intake, during the last 3 weeks of which they underwent a second metabolic balance study. Both parenteral and oral intake combined were calculated to maintain a total intake of greater than 75 cal/kg/day for 6 to 8 weeks. Patients were then sent home during Period III for 5 weeks on customary diet and activity. They subsequently returned to the hospital for a final 3 week balance study.

Results of the study are summarized here. The patients ranged in age from 9 to 17 years (mean 14 years) and had a height age ranging from 6 to 10 years, a weight age ranging from 6 to 12 years, and a bone age delay of 2 to 5 years behind chronological age (mean 3 years). Symptoms had been present for an average of 6 years (range 2 to 8 years) prior to study, and growth failure had been present for an average of 5 years (range 1 to 8 years) prior to study. Height age and weight age were very close, reflecting the fact that, although short, the patients were of normal pro-

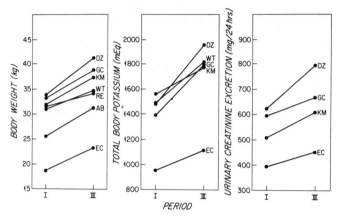

**Figure 2.** Body composition before and after nutritional therapy for Crohn's disease. Note change in body weight (left), total body potassium (middle), and creatinine excretion (right). Data were obtained before and after combined oral and parenteral intake averaging 75 kcal/ kg/ day.

portion. Six of the seven patients were prepubertal; the other was at Tanner stage III but had amenorrhea. No patient had clinical symptoms of gastrointestinal disease during the study, and four were on stable doses of prednisone not exceeding 20 mg/day throughout the study period.

Included in the baseline observations made in Period I were standard evaluations of absorptive function by 72 hour fecal fat excretion, xylose absorption, and serum folic acid, carotene, and vitamin $B_{12}$ levels, all of which were either normal or minimally deranged. The only abnormalities that were present at the start of the study, and persisted, were elevated sedimentation rates and mildly abnormal [51]chromium-labeled albumin excretion in the stool (not exceeding 3%). Endocrine function in the patients studied was also normal, including plasma somatomedin levels (kindly performed by Dr. Lewis Underwood and Judson VanWyck). Basal metabolic rates when compared to normal values for height age were also normal, strongly suggesting that energy expenditures were not increased by inflammatory disease.

When the daily caloric intake for all of the patients was measured and compared to normal data obtained from the monograph of McCammon and co-workers (31), it was clear that in Period I, our patients' caloric intake averaged 82 ± 17% of the normal values for height age. During Period II, parenteral nutrition increased the mean intake to 136 ± 21% of caloric requirements, and after cessation of nutritional support in

Table 6    Growth Response to Nutritional Support in Crohn's Disease

| Patient | Age at Onset of Treatment (yrs) | Cumulative Height at Follow-up[a] (cm) |
|---------|---------------------------------|----------------------------------------|
| EC | 9.3 | 6.0 (1) |
| WT | 11.3 | 7.0 (1) |
| KM | 12.3 | 6.5 (1) |
| RE | 15.1 | 13.6 (3) |
| AB | 15.2 | 22.0 (3) |
| GC | 15.8 | 3.0 (3) |
| DZ | 17.0 | 10.0 (3) |

[a] Number in ( ) is time of follow-up.

Period III, there was a decrease to 78 ± 20% of required calories for height age. The changes in total body weight in seven patients, lean body mass in five patients and creatinine production in four patients were studied from Period I to Period III (Figure 2). There was a marked increase in body weight in response to therapy, accompanied by a corresponding increase in total body potassium and creatinine excretion. These data indicate that a significant proportion of total body weight accrued was lean body mass and muscle mass. Data for nitrogen balance (not shown) indicated that three patients were in nitrogen balance prior to therapy and their nitrogen retention increased significantly in response to increased nutritional support. One patient was in negative nitrogen balance in Period I and had only a small, though statistically significant, increase in nitrogen retention during therapy.

Dramatic and sustained acceleration in growth velocity occurred in response to therapy. Height response data for individual patients are shown in Table 6. Cumulative growth was from 3 to 22 cm at 1 to 3 years following intravenous hyperalimentation. All patients began to grow during therapy. Patient G.C., who was the only pubescent patient at the time of the study, grew only 3 centimeters in 3 years. The most likely explanation for this blunted response was her advanced development. In fact, she had already attained 97% of her projected adult height as estimated from the data of Bayer and Bayley (32). The other patients all showed a return of growth rate to normal levels. If sustained, these growth patterns would have returned the patients to their premorbid growth channel. However, with cessation of total parenteral nutrition, nutritional intake decreased, as recorded above, and the growth rate fell in parallel. Nevertheless, it was clear that correcting the deficits acquired during the onset of growth failure appeared to have allowed temporary restitution of normal growth rates.

Using supplemental oral nutritional support, Kirschner and co-workers (33) have reported stimulation of growth in children with Crohn's disease and growth retardation. All of these patients had active intestinal disease. Growth velocity in three of the seven patients rose from 2.5 cm before to 5 to 6 cm/year during therapy.

Thus:

1. Growth failure in Crohn's disease is usually accompanied by a markedly reduced caloric intake.
2. In our patients, abnormal growth was unrelated to malabsorption, significant intestinal protein loss, steroid effects, or endocrine dysfunction.
3. The normal metabolic rate in the patients studied indicated that the energy cost of disease was not increased.
4. Caloric supplementation begun immediately at the time growth failure is first noticed may be adequate to prevent prolonged effects of Crohn's disease on growth.
5. If oral supplementation with an elemental formula fails, central venous parenteral nutrition has been shown by our studies to increase lean body mass and induce linear growth.
6. Dramatic and prolonged increases in linear growth can be achieved by these techniques and this provides a new approach to the treatment of growth failure in inflammatory bowel disease. It is possible that to be maximally effective, therapy must be instituted before puberty.

In clinical management of patients with inflammatory bowel disease, the primary goal is to identify the earliest possible state of nutritional failure and to institute appropriate nutritional support and supplementation before the impact of malnutrition becomes manifest. Using this approach, it should be possible in the future to prevent the serious complications of malnutrition so common in inflammatory bowel disease today.

## ACKNOWLEDGMENTS

The author is indebted to many colleagues who have contributed to this work: Drs. Drew G. Kelts, Kon-Taik Khaw, John B. Watkins, Warren E. Grupe, John F. Crigler, Grace Shen, Steven L. Werlin; Ms. Carol Boehme, Ms. Meryl Adler, and Mr. Ian Barwick.

# REFERENCES

1. P. Razen, J. Zonis, P. Yekutiel, et al., Crohn's disease in the Jewish population of Tel-Aviv-Yafo, *Gastroenterology*, **76**, 25 (1979).

2. A. L. Mendeloff, "The Epidemiology of Idiopathic Inflammatory Bowel Disease," in J. B. Kirsner and R. G. Shorter, Eds., *Inflammatory Bowel Disease*, Lea and Febiger, Philadelphia, 1975, pp. 3–22.

3. H. Schachter and J. B. Kirsner, Definition of inflammatory bowel disease of unknown etiology, *Gastroenterology*, **68**, 591 (1975).

4. A. N. Smith and T. W. Balfour, "Malabsorption in Crohn's Disease," in B. N. Brooke, Ed., *Clinics in Gastroenterology: Crohn's Disease*, Saunders, London, 1972, pp. 433–448.

5. W. Beeken, H. J. Busch, and D. L. Sylvester, Intestinal protein loss in Crohn's disease, *Gastroenterology*, **62**, 207 (1972).

6. W. Beeken, Absorptive defects in young people with regional enteritis, *Pediatrics*, **52**, 69 (1973).

7. C. D. Gerson, N. Cohen, and H. J. Janowitz, Small intestinal absorptive function in regional enteritis, *Gastroenterology*, **64**, 907 (1973).

8. W. L. Beeken and R. E. Kanich, Microbial flora of the upper small bowel in Crohn's disease, *Gastroenterology*, **65**, 390 (1973).

9. E. L. Krawitt, W. L. Beeken, and C. D. Janney, Calcium absorption in Crohn's disease, *Gastroenterology*, **71**, 251 (1976).

10. R. W. Wannemacher, Jr., "Protein Metabolism," in H. Ghadimi, Ed., *Total Parenteral Nutrition*, Wiley, New York, 1975, pp. 85–153.

11. M. Berger, D. Gribetz, and B. I. Korelitz, Growth retardation in children with ulcerative colitis: the effect of medical and surgical therapy, *Pediatrics*, **55**, 459 (1975).

12. D. R. Homer, P. J. Grand, and A. H. Colodny, Growth, course and prognosis after surgery for Crohn's disease, *Pediatrics*, **59**, 717 (1977).

13. P. F. Whittington, H. V. Barnes, and T. M. Bayless, Medical management of Crohn's disease in adolescence, *Gastroenterology*, **72**, 1338 (1977).

14. D. G. Kelts, R. J. Grand, G. Shen, J. B. Watkins, S. L. Werlin, and C. Boehme, Nutritional basis of growth failure in children and adolescents with Crohn's disease. *Gastroenterology* (1979) (in press).

15. E. Lebenthal, I. Antonowicz, and H. Schwachman, Correlation of lactase activity and lactose tolerance and milk consumption in different age groups, *Am. J. Clin. Nutr.*, **28**, 595 (1975).

16. N. W. Solomons, R. L. Rosenfield, R. A. Jacob, et al., Growth retardation and zinc nutrition, *Pediat. Res.*, **10**, 923 (1976).

17. K. Gerlach, D. A. Morowitz, and J. B. Kirsner, Symptomatic hypomagnesemia complicating regional enteritis, *Gastroenterology*, **59**, 567 (1970).

18. R. J. Grand and A. H. Colodny, Increased requirement for magnesium during parenteral therapy for granulomatous colitis, *J. Pediat.* **8**, 788 (1972).

19. R. J. Grand and D. R. Homer, Approaches to inflammatory bowel disease in childhood and adolescence, *Pediat. Clin. N.A.*, **22**, 835 (1975).

20. T. D. McCaffery, K. Nasr, A. H. Lawrence, et al., Severe growth retardation in children with inflammatory bowel disease. *J. Pediat.*, **45**, 386 (1970).

21. J. C. Waterlow, Classification and definition of protein calorie malnutrition, *Brit. Med. J.*, **2**, 566 (1972).

22. D. B. Grant, J. Hambley, D. J. Becker, et al., Reduced sulphation factors in undernourished children, *Arch. Dis. Childh.*, **48**, 596 (1973).

23. A. Prader, J. M. Tanner, and G. A. Von Harnack, Catch-up growth following illness or starvation, *J. Pediat.*, **62**, 646 (1963).

24. G. B. Forbes, A note on the mathematics of catch-up growth, *Pediat. Res.*, **8**, 929 (1974).

25. H. L. Green, A. E. Slonim, J. A. O'Neill, et al., Continuous nocturnal intragastric feeding for management of glycogen storage disease, *New Engl. J. Med.*, **294**, 423 (1976).

26. J. E. Fisher, G. S. Foster, R. M. Abel, et al., Hyperalimentation as primary therapy for inflammatory bowel disease, *Am. J. Surg.*, **125**, 165 (1973).

27. D. L. Anderson and H. W. Boyce, Use of parenteral nutrition in treatment of advanced regional enteritis, *Am. J. Dig. Dis.*, **18**, 633 (1973).

28. C. M. Vogel, T. R. Corwin, and A. E. Baue, Intravenous hyperalimentation in the treatment of inflammatory diseases of the bowel, *Arch. Surg.*, **108**, 460 (1974).

29. A. Tenore, W. F. Berman, J. S. Parks, et al., Basal and stimulated growth hormone concentrations in inflammatory bowel disease, *J. Clin. Endocrinol. Metab.*, **44**, 622 (1977).

30. T. D. McCaffery, K. Nasr, A. M. Lawrence, et al., Effect of administered human growth hormone on growth retardation in inflammatory bowel disease, *Am. J. Dig. Dis.*, **19**, 411 (1974).

31. R. W. McCammon, *Human Growth and Development*, Charles Thomas, Springfield, Illinois, 1970, pp. 63–100.

32. L. M. Bayer and N. Bayley, *Growth Diagnosis*, 2nd ed., University of Chicago Press, Chicago, Ill., 1976, pp. 214–233.

33. B. Kirschner, O. Voinchet, and I. H. Rosenberg, Growth retardation in inflammatory bowel disease, *Gastroenterology*, **75**, 504 (1978).

# 9

## Peptic Ulcer: Epidemiology, Nutritional Aspects, Drugs, Smoking, Alcohol, and Diet

JON I. ISENBERG, M.D.

VA Wadsworth Medical Center, Los Angeles, California, and the UCLA School of Medicine, Los Angeles, California.

### EPIDEMIOLOGY

The marked epidemiological changes that have occurred in peptic ulcer disease make studying the nutritional aspects of peptic ulcer difficult (1). According to the best available information, prior to the 18th century, peptic ulcer disease was infrequent (2). In the 19th century, gastric ulcer was many times more common than duodenal ulcer, the latter being a rare disease. During this century, there have been marked changes in the apparent incidence of duodenal ulcer (3). Specifically, duodenal ulcer was uncommon at the turn of the century, and reached a peak incidence in Great Britain during the 1950s. The cohort born between 1885 and 1895 had the highest death rate due to duodenal ulcer disease; the reason for this is not known (4). From 1958 until 1972, there has been a progressive decrease in the number of hospital admissions for both duodenal and gastric ulcer (both perforated and nonperforated) (5). It is assumed that those patients who have a perforated ulcer are admitted to a hospital, and thereby reflect the prevalence of ulcer disease within the general population. It is not known whether this is a valid assumption. Also, the ratio of duodenal ulcer in males to females has decreased drastically. In 1928, the ratio of perforated duodenal ulcer in males to females was 19 to 1. In 1967, this ratio had decreased to 5 to 1 (6). The explanation for the apparent decreased incidence of ulcer disease in men with a less

141

marked decrease in females, is not known. It is also not known whether the incidence of ulcer disease has decreased, or whether there has been a decrease in the severity of ulcer disease, or a combination of both.

The cumulative lifetime incidence of duodenal ulcer in males in the United States, as estimated by Monson and MacMahon, was approximately 12%, and 1.5% for gastric ulcer (7). The incidence of duodenal ulcer in males is estimated at about 2 per 1000 adults per year, and in females, about 0.8 per 1000 adults per year (8). The incidence of gastric ulcer in males is estimated at about 0.3 per 1000 adults per year and in females, approximately 0.3 per 1000 per year (9). According to Bonnevie, the "symptomatic debut" of duodenal ulcer peaks in males at about age 20 to 30, and in females, at age 40 to 50 (8). The "symptomatic debut" of gastric ulcer peaks in both males and females at about age 50 to 60 (9).

## NUTRITIONAL ASPECTS

The precise role of nutritional factors in the pathogenesis of peptic ulcer are far from fully understood. There have been only a few experimental studies, and there is even less information available in man. In the 1920s and 1930s, studies in animals indicated that partial or total starvation produced gastric ulcers (10–12). In rats, experimental gastric ulcer formation could be prevented by feeding either oral glucose or other food substances (13). Two separate groups demonstrated that either a diet low in protein, or an almost protein-free diet, produced juxtapyloric ulcers in approximately 50% of dogs tested (14–15).

The mechanism of partial starvation-induced, or total starvation-induced ulcer formation has not been fully defined. Interestingly, Enochs and co-workers recently confirmed the observation that all dextrose prevented gastric stress ulcers in rats (16). A series of experiments by Menguy and associates examined gastric mucosal cellular function in rabbits and rats subjected to hypovolemia-induced stress ulcers (17–20). Their studies revealed the following findings:

1. Hypovolemic shock produced a prompt and significant decrease in gastric mucosal ATP, ADP, and total adenosine phosphates.
2. Glucagon stores, which are minimal in the gastric mucosa, were further diminished in the presence of hypovolemic shock.
3. The decrease in oxidative phosphorylation that occurred during shock was significantly greater in the gastric corpus when compared to the gastric antrum. This corresponds to the location of stress ulcers, which occur almost entirely within the gastric corpus.

4. Feeding tended to prevent the corpus lesions and, importantly, decreased the changes that occurred in high-energy phosphates.

Taken together, these observations suggest that stress-induced gastric ulcers in animals can be prevented by oral glucose. The role of protein, fat, or both in preventing these lesions has not been studied. Second, the stress-induced ulcers may be related to changes in cellular high-energy phosphate metabolism. Finally, since stress-induced ulceration in man is an important clinical problem with both a high morbidity and a high mortality, clinical studies are needed to contrast the role of oral glucose versus other foodstuffs and appropriate controls in preventing stress ulcers in man.

The role of vitamin deficiency in ulcerogenesis also is not fully clarified. A number of years ago, experimental studies suggested that deficiencies of either vitamin A, thiamine, or vitamin B complex could produce ulcers in experimental animals (21). There is no apparent clinical counterpart of vitamin deficiency resulting in peptic ulcer.

The role of nutrition in human peptic ulcer has also not been carefully studied. Epidemiological studies in India indicate that peptic ulcer (both gastric and duodenal ulcer) is more common in the south than in the north. This has been attributed by Malhotra to marked dietary differences (22). The diet in the south of India contains largely defined carbohydrates in large quantities of liquids, and hence does not require mastication. The diet in the north is a thick diet, requiring thorough mastication and mixing with saliva. Malhotra postulated that the more rapidly eaten liquid diet, in the absence of adequate salivation, predisposes to ulcer formation. This hypothesis may have some merit in that epidermal growth factor–urogastrone is excreted by the salivary glands (23). Urogastrone has recently been demonstrated to be a potent inhibitor of pentagastrin-stimulated gastric acid secretion in man, and to expedite the healing of experimental gastric ulcers in rats (24, 25). Additional studies are badly needed to correlate the urogastrone production in man with diet, and with the development of peptic ulcer.

Although there are distinct geographical differences in diet and in the incidence of ulcer, there are no recognized causal relationships between the dietary differences in ulcer incidence. During the two World Wars, there were no clear-cut changes in ulcer incidence that could be related to changes in nutritional status alone. During World War I the incidence of gastric and duodenal ulcer was low. During World War II the incidence of ulcer in United States troops overseas was 1.4 to 2.3 per 1000 per year, compared to an incidence in the United States of 2.5 to 4.2 per 1000 per year. Therefore, there was no evidence of an increased incidence of ulcer disease in the United States troops who were overseas, and probably subjected to a less nutritious diet. There was an increase in ulcer disease, particularly during the early part of World War II, in England, Sweden, Norway, and Switzerland (26). Whether this increase was principally of nutritional origin, or whether it was related to the multitude of other effects produced by the war is not known.

In summary, there is no clear-cut information that incriminates malnutrition, either of vitamins or of nutrients, with peptic ulcer disease in man. Two areas that deserve further exploration in man are:

1. The role of oral glucose, and other nutrients, in preventing stress-induced lesions.
2. The secretion and role of urogastrone–epidermal growth factor in preventing ulceration and expediting the healing of ulcers, and its secretory rate in relation to the prevalence of ulcer.

## DRUGS

Cooke has thoroughly reviewed the association of drugs and peptic ulcer (27). These studies can be summarized as follows: First, to demonstrate either an increased or a decreased prevalence of drug-related ulcer disease, there should be two identical study populations, one treated with the drug in question and the other treated with placebo. Few such studies have been conducted, and the reference, or control, population has often been the prevalence of ulcer disease in the general population as a whole.

Second, aspirin has been established beyond doubt to be associated with the development of gastric ulcer. Levy reported that the incidence of hospital-diagnosed aspirin-induced gastric ulcers was approximately 14 per 100,000 population per year in those who were taking aspirin regularly at least 4 or more days per week, as compared with four per 100,000 in those who did not use aspirin (28). The mechanism of aspirin-induced ulcer formation is not fully understood; however, it may be related to two identified factors:

1. Aspirin is known to damage the gastric mucosal barrier to hydrogen ion, and thereby to permit back diffusion of hydrogen ion into the mucosa (29).
2. Aspirin inhibits the production of prostaglandins (30). Many prostaglandins have been shown to protect the gastric mucosa from a large number of exogenous factors that are capable of producing damage

(31). The aspirin-induced decrease in prostaglandins may be instrumental in ulcer formation.

Third, as I interpret the data, there is an association between aspirin ingestion and upper gastrointestinal hemorrhage, either hematemesis or melena. The results of eight studies that compared aspirin intake in hospitalized patients with upper gastrointestinal bleeding to intake in a similar hospitalized patient population without upper gastrointestinal bleeding revealed that 406 of 814 patients (49.8%) with upper GI bleeding had a history of aspirin ingestion, while 318 of 1111 hospitalized nonbleeding patients (28.6%) had a history of recent aspirin intake, a highly significant difference (27). The percentage of aspirin ingestors in the patients with GI bleeding ranged from 33 to 68% in the various studies, compared to aspirin intake in the GI nonbleeders ranging from 4 to 46%. Also, the site of gastrointestinal bleeding in aspirin ingestors tends to be acute gastric erosions, rather than chronic peptic ulcer. Levy also noted an increased prevalence of upper gastrointestinal bleeding in patients who consumed aspirin at least 4 days per week (28). Interestingly, the difference was not apparent in patients with newly diagnosed duodenal ulcer or in patients who consumed aspirin fewer than 4 days per week.

Fourth, indomethacin, phenylbutazone, and other nonsteroidal anti-inflammatory agents have not been adequately studied to draw any meaningful conclusions about whether they were associated with peptic ulcer or gastrointestinal bleeding. Indomethacin has similar effects to aspirin, and theoretically should produce similar untoward clinical effects (32). Only additional studies designed to contrast ulcer prevalence and gastrointestinal bleeding in patients treated with these agents with an appropriate control group will shed light on this important clinical area.

Fifth, the role of corticosteroids in ulcer pathogenesis is not, and probably never will be, fully understood. This is largely because there will not be adequately large samples treated in double-blind, prospective, controlled fashion in diseases where steroids have been of proven efficacy. However, Conn and Blitzer reviewed 6102 patients who were studied in 32 double-blind and 18 nondouble-blind studies (33). Their data can be interpreted in two ways. Corticosteroids can produce ulcer or an exacerbation of ulcer disease in patients who are treated with steroids for more than 30 days, or with a high total dose of corticosteroids for more than 30 days, or with a high total dose of corticosteroids equivalent to 1000 mg of prednisone, and in patients with a prior history of ulcer. Also, the results indicate that short duration (less than 30 days), low total dose (less than 1000 mg of prednisone), and ACTH, were not associated with an increased prevalence of ulcer. There was no evidence that steroids were associated with upper gastrointestinal hemorrhage, superficial gastric erosions, or ulcer symptoms. It therefore appears that in those circumstances which require high total dose of steroids, or a long duration of treatment, or in those patients with a prior history of ulcer, steroids may be instrumental in either ulcer formation or reactivation.


## SMOKING

There is a distinct relation between cigarette smoking and peptic ulcer disease both in males and in females. This has been reviewed (34). The incidence of both gastric and duodenal ulcer is greater in cigarette smokers than in nonsmokers (7, 35). There also appears to be a direct relationship between ulcer prevalence and number of cigarettes smoked per day, duration of smoking history, and inhalation of tobacco (36). The ratio of peptic ulcer in smokers to nonsmokers is approximately 1.8. Therefore, a cigarette smoker is about twice as likely to develop an ulcer as a nonsmoker.

There is evidence which suggests that discontinuing smoking expedites ulcer healing (37). However, it is not possible to conduct an ideal study in this area, since physicians can only recommend to the patient that he or she stop smoking, but many continue to smoke. In spite of this, there is a suggestion that in those patients who discontinue smoking ulcer healing is more rapid than in those who continue to smoke (37). In addition, morbidity and mortality due to ulcer is about two times greater in those patients who smoke than in their nonsmoking ulcer counterparts (38). The mechanisms by which cigarette smoking affects ulcer pathogenesis or healing are not fully understood. Smoking does not affect gastric acid or pepsin secretion (39). However, recent evidence indicates that smoking decreased secretin-stimulated pancreatic bicarbonate secretion, a factor that may play a role in the pathogenesis of duodenal ulcer (40). Smoking has also been demonstrated to decrease the resting pyloric sphincter pressure in man (41), increase duodenogastric reflux (42), and slow gastric emptying (43), factors that may be important in the pathogenesis of gastric ulcer.


## ALCOHOL

Although alcohol ingestion is often discouraged in patients with peptic ulcer disease, there is no definite scientific basis for this recommendation

(27). First, although alcohol slightly stimulates gastric secretion in dogs, it does not increase gastric acid secretion in man (44). Second, there are no epidemiological data which indicate that alcohol ingestion is associated with an increased risk of peptic ulcer disease (36). In fact, a number of studies have failed to demonstrate an association between alcohol intake and peptic ulcer. The only indirect association between alcohol and peptic ulcer is in those patients who have established alcoholic cirrhosis, where there tends to be an increased prevalence of ulcer disease (45).

## DIET

In spite of the lack of evidence that a bland diet alters ulcer symptoms, healing rate, recurrences, or complications, a bland diet is still the most commonly used diet in hospitalized patients with peptic ulcer. In a recent survey of 326 hospitals representing 12% of the hospital beds in the United States, 250 (77%) prescribed a bland diet for patients with peptic ulcer (46). Ten percent of hospitals prescribed a "sippy diet", and only 6% prescribed a regular diet. Since a bland diet and a regular diet produce similar stimulation of gastric acid secretion, there is no physiologic basis for prescribing a bland diet in the treatment of patients with peptic ulcer. Also, frequent feedings, or hourly milk, have been demonstrated to produce a lower gastric pH (i.e., a higher gastric acidity) than three regular meals per day (47). This is, as one might anticipate, the result of the continuous stimulatory effect of frequent feedings as compared to three meals per day.

Although milk has been shown to be an important stimulus of gastric acid secretion from 2 to 4 hours after its ingestion, milk was prescribed as part of ulcer patients' treatment in 57% of hospitals surveyed, with a mean daily intake of 32 ounces (46). Also, about half of the hospitals recommend that the patients ingest some form of bland diet after they are discharged. A single glass of milk has been demonstrated to increase gastric secretion in duodenal ulcer patients to about 30% of maximal histamine-stimulated acid secretion (48). Also, there is some suggestive evidence that coronary artery disease is more prevalent in patients who have been treated with an ulcer diet containing large quantities of milk. For example, the mortality rate from arteriosclerotic heart disease was approximately 1.5 times greater in subjects with ulcer disease than in the general population (45). Whether this is related to the ulcer diet, or to the association of one disease with another, or to other unrecognizable factors, is not fully understood. Also, the frequent ingestion of milk when combined with calcium-containing antacids can produce hypercalcemia and impaired renal function. In summary, milk is not recommended as routine form of therapy in patients with peptic ulcer because its buffering effect is only transient, and it is a potent stimulus of gastric secretion after it has left the stomach.

Avoidance of spices, fruit juices, coffee, and alcohol has been recommended frequently for patients with peptic ulcer. There is no evidence to indicate that any one of these affects ulcer healing, complications, or recurrences one way or the other (49). The effects of these agents on these parameters of ulcer disease have been inadequately studied. Interestingly, regular coffee and decaffeinated coffee stimulate gastric acid secretion equally (50), and as mentioned above, alcohol does not stimulate gastric acid secretion and in fact may produce slight suppression. Although coffee ingestion during college has been suggested as a possible factor in ulcer development in later life (51), in a retrospective study of 36,656 patients, Friedman and co-workers were unable to demonstrate an association either between coffee intake (six or more cups per day) or alcohol ingestion with an increased prevalence of ulcer (36).

In summary, there are many myths regarding diet and peptic ulcer. At present, there is no evidence that any specific foodstuffs are associated with the development of ulcer. Neither is there any evidence that the avoidance of any specific foodstuffs affects the rate of ulcer healing or its complications. It is therefore recommended that the ulcer patient be placed on a regular diet.

## THE FUTURE

There are a number of areas related to the role of nutrition and ulcerogenesis which deserve further study. In the area of experimental formation, these include: (1) the importance of individual and mixed vitamin deficiencies; (2) the role of urogastrone (its secretion, metabolic affects, and its role in the prevention of experimental ulcer); (3) the mechanisms involved in protein deprivation-induced experimental ulcers in dogs; and (4) the role of high-energy phosphate metabolism in other types of experimentally induced ulcer formation. In addition, there are a number of clinical areas that require further study. These include: (1) carefully controlled clinical trials that examine the role of spices, alcohol, and caffeine intake on ulcer healing rates, complications, and recurrences; (2) the role of indomethacin and other nonsteroidal anti-inflammatory agents in the development of gastric ulcers, as well as their effects on upper gastrointestinal bleeding; and (3) carefully obtained nutritional intake histories in large population groups that are currently being studied for ulcer (e.g., Kaiser-Permanente, and Rand Health Care Delivery Systems) for the identification of discrete nutritional differences between patients with ulcer and normal subjects.

## REFERENCES

1. R. A. L. Sturdevant, Epidemiology of peptic ulcer: Report of a conference, *Am. J. Epidemiol.*, **104**, 9 (1976).
2. J. Abercrombie, *Diseases of the Stomach*, Murray, London, 1830.
3. A. I. Mendeloff, What has been happening to duodenal ulcer?, *Gastroenterology*, **67**, 1020 (1974).
4. M. Susser, Causes of peptic ulcer; A selective epidemiologic review, *J. Chron. Dis.* **20**, 435 (1967).
5. R. C. Brown, M. J. S. Langman, and P. M. Lambert, Hospital admissions for peptic ulcer during 1958–1972, *Brit. Med. J.*, **1**, 35 (1976).
6. M. Langman, "The Changing Nature of Duodenal Ulcer Diathesis," in, Westminster Hospital Symposium on Chronic Duodenal Ulcer, Buttersworth, London, 1974, p. 3.
7. R. R. Monson and B. MacMahon, Peptic ulcer in Massachusetts physicians, *New Engl. J. Med.*, **281**, 11 (1969).
8. O. Bonnevie, The incidence of gastric ulcer in Copenhagen County, *Scand. J. Gastroent.*, **10**, 231 (1975).
9. O. Bonnevie, The incidence of duodenal ulcer in Copenhagen County, *Scand. J. Gatsroent.*, **10**, 385 (1975).
10. A. M. Pappenheimer and L. D. Larimore, Occurrence of gastric lesions in rats: Their relation to dietary deficiency and hair ingestion, *J. Exper. Med.*, **40**, 719 (1924).
11. H. E. Magee, W. Anderson, and J. McCallum, Diet and peptic ulcer in cavies, *Lancet*, **1**, 12 (1929).
12. F. Hoelzel and E. DaCosta, Production of ulcers in the prostomach of rats by protein restriction, *Proc. Soc. Exper. Biol. Med.*, **29**, 382 (1931).
13. C. K. Chen, Experimental gastric ulcer in albino rats, *Am. J. Dig. Dis.*, **8**, 28 (1941).
14. A. A. Weech and B. H. Paige, Nutritional edema in the dog: IV. Peptic ulcer produced by the same low protein diet that leads to hypoproteinemia and edema, *Am. J. Path.*, **13**, 249, (1937).
15. T. Li and S. Freeman, The frequency of "peptic ulcer" in protein deficient dogs, *Gastroenterology*, **6**, 140 (1946).
16. M. R. Enochs, J. England, and K. J. Ivey, Dextrose protection against stress lesions in rats: Relationship to insulin and glucagon, *Gastroenterology*, **74**, 1032 (1978).
17. R. Menguy, L. Desbaillets, and Y. F. Masters, Mechanism of stress ulcer: Influence of hypovolemic shock on energy metabolism in the gastric mucosa, *Gastroenterology*, **66**, 46 (1974).

18. R. Menguy and Y. F. Masters, Mechanism of stress ulcer. II Differences between the antrum, corpus, and fundus with respect to the effects of complete ischemia on gastric mucosal energy metabolism, *Gastroenterology*, **66**, 509 (1974).

19. R. Menguy and Y. F. Masters, Mechanism of stress ulcer. III. Effects of hemorrhagic shock on energy metabolism in the mucosa of the antrum, corpus, and fundus of the rabbit stomach, *Gastroenterology*, **66**, 1168 (1974).

20. R. Menguy and Y. F. Masters, Mechanism of stress ulcer IV. Influence of fasting on the tolerance of gastric mucosal energy metabolism to ischemia and on the incidence of stress ulceration, *Gastroenterology*, **66**, 1177 (1974).

21. A. C. Ivy, M. I. Grossman, and W. H. Bachrach, *Peptic Ulcer, 1950*, Blakiston, Philadelphia and Toronto, pp. 306–313.

22. S. L. Malhotra, Peptic ulcer in India and its aetiology, *Gut*, **5**, 412 (1964).

23. H. Gregory, Isolation and structure of urogastrone and its relationship to epidermal growth factor, *Nature* (Lond.), **257**, 325 (1975).

24. J. B. Elder, P. C. Ganguli, I. E. Gillespie, et al., Effect of urogastrone on gastric secretion and plasma gastrin levels in normal subjects, *Gut*, **16**, 887 (1975).

25. C. G. Koffman, J. Berry, and J. B. Elder, A comparison of cimetidine and epidermal growth factor in the healing of experimental gastric ulcers, *Brit. J. Sup.* **64**, 830 (1977).

26. A. C. Ivy, M. I. Grossman, and W. H. Bachrach, *Peptic Ulcer, 1950*, Blakiston, Philadelphia and Toronto, pp. 660–664.

27. A. R. Cooke, "Drug Damage to the Gastroduodenum," in *Gastrointestinal Disease*, 2nd Ed., Saunders, Philadelphia, 1978, Volume I.

28. M. Levy, Aspirin use in patients with major upper gastrointestinal bleeding and peptic-ulcer disease, *New Engl. J. Med.*, **290**, 1158 (1974).

29. H. W. Davenport, Salicylate damage to the gastric mucosal barrier, *New Engl. J. Med.*, **276**, 1307 (1967).

30. J. R. Vane, Inhibition of prostaglandin synthesis as a mechanism of action for aspirin-like drugs, *Nature New Biol.*, **231–232**, 1971.

31. A. Robert, Antisecretory, antiulcer, cytoprotective and diarrheogenic properties of prostaglandins, in B. Samuelson and R. Paoletti, Eds., *Advances in Prostaglandin and Thromboxane Research*, Raven Press, New York, 1975, pp. 507–520.

32. B. P. Maclaurin, D. A. Richards, and D. Heads, Indomethacin associated gastric and duodenal ulceration. Presented at the Annual Meeting of the N.Z. Society of Gastroenterology, September, 1977.

33. H. O. Conn and B. L. Blitzer, Medical progress: Nonassociation of adrenocorticosteroid therapy and peptic ulcer, *New Engl. J. Med.*, **294**, 473 (1976).

34. A. Harrison, J. Elashoff, and M. I. Grossman, "Cigarette Smoking and Ulcer Disease," in *The Surgeon General's Report on Smoking and Health*, 1979 edition (in press).

35. A. Kasanen and J. Forsstrom, Social stress and living habits in the etiology of peptic ulcer, *Ann. Med. Int. Fen.* **55**, 13 (1966).

36. G. D. Friedman, A. B. Siegelaub, C. C. Seltzer, Cigarettes, alcohol, coffee and peptic ulcer, *New. Engl. J. Med.*, **290**, 469 (1974).

37. R. Doll, F. Jones, and F. Pygott, Effect of smoking on the production and maintenance of gastric and duodenal ulcers, *Lancet*, **1**, 657 (1958).

38. E. C. Hammond and D. Horn, Smoking and death rates—Report on forty-four months of follow-up of 187,783 men, *J.A.M.A.*, **166**, 1294 (1958).

39. W. P. Fung and C. Y. Tye, Effect of smoking on gastric acid secretion, *Aust. and New Zeal. J. Med.*, **3**, 251 (1973).

40. S. Murthy, V. Dinoso, H. Clearfield, and W. Chey, Simultaneous measurement of basal pancreatic, gastric acid secretion, plasma gastrin, and secretin during smoking, *Gastroenterology*, **73**, 758 (1977).

41. J. Valenzuela, C. Defilippi, and A. Csendes, Manometric studies on the human pyloric sphincter, *Gastroenterology*, **70**, 481 (1976).

42. N. W. Read and P. Grech, Effect of cigarette smoking on competence of the pylorus: preliminary study, *Brit. Med. J.*, **3**, 313 (1973).

43. D. S. Grimes and J. Goddard, Effect of cigarette smoking on gastric emptying, *Brit. Med. J.*, **2**, 460 (1978).

44. A. R. Cooke, Ethanol and gastric function, *Gastroenterology*, **62**, 501 (1972).

45. M. J. S. Langman and A. R. Cooke, Gastric and duodenal ulcer and the associated diseases, *Lancet*, **1**, 680 (1976).

46. J. Welsh, Diet therapy of peptic ulcer disease, *Gastroenterology*, **72**, 740, (1977).

47. J. B. Kirsner and W. L. Palmer, The effect of various antacids on the hydrogen ion concentration of the gastric contents, *Am. J. Dig. Dis.*, **7**, 85 (1940).

48. A. F. Ippoliti, V. A. Maxwell, and J. I. Isenberg, The effect of various forms of milk on gastric acid secretion. Studies in patients with duodenal ulcer and normal subjects, *Ann. Int. Med.*, **84**, 286 (1976).

49. W. L. Peterson and J. S. Fordtran, *Reduction of Gastric Acidity*, in *Gastrointestinal Disease*, 2nd Ed., Vol. 1, Saunders, Philadelphia, 1978, p. 891.

50. S. Cohen and G. H. Barth, Gastric acid secretion and lower-esophagealsphincter pressure in response to coffee and caffeine, *New Engl. J. Med.*, **293**, 897 (1975).

51. D. J. Sandweiss, The sippy treatment for peptic ulcer—fifty years later, *Am. J. Dig. Dis.*, **6**, 929 (1961).

# 10

## Alcohol, Nutrition, and Liver Disease

CHARLES S. LIEBER, M.D.

Veterans Administration Hospital, Bronx, New York, and Mount Sinai School of Medicine of the City University of New York

Malnutrition and alcoholism are commonly associated. Thirty years ago researchers considered the possibility that malnutrition promotes alcoholism. More recently, this theory has been abandoned. Malnutrition, including impaired digestion and absorption, is now considered a result of chronic alcohol consumption. Alcohol and nutrition interact at many levels (Table 1). Ethanol may directly alter the level of nutrient intake by reducing appetite, by displacing food in the diet, or by virtue of its deleterious effects at almost every level of the gastrointestinal tract, which result in disturbances of digestion and absorption. Furthermore, through its effect on various organs, especially the liver, ethanol may alter the transport, activation, catabolism, utilization, and storage of almost every nutrient studied. Therefore, alcoholism remains one of the major causes of nutritional deficiency syndromes in our society. Furthermore, ethanol is directly toxic to many tissues of the body and this effect may be potentiated by concomitant nutritional deficiencies. Thus, because of its widespread use and multiple effects, ethanol has a major impact on the overall nutritional status.

Many of the original studies summarized here were supported by grants from the National Institute of Alcohol Abuse and Alcoholism, the National Institute of Arthritis, Metabolism, and Digestive Diseases, and the Medical Research Service of the Veterans Administration.

## Table 1    Alcohol-Nutrition Interaction

1. Primary malnutrition (deficient intake)
   a. "Empty" calories
   b. Economic factors
   c. Impared appetite secondary to GI-liver disorders
2. Secondary malnutrition (deficient nutrient utilization)
   a. Ethanol-induced GI damage (maldigestion-malabsorption)
   b. Deficiency-induced intestinal dysfunction
   c. Energy wastage
   d. Decreased activation or increased inactivation of nutrients

## EFFECTS OF ALCOHOL ABUSE ON THE GASTROINTESTINAL TRACT

Ethanol may affect the stomach in a number of ways. Acid secretion may be increased as a result of direct stimulation, vagal effects, or through gastrin release (1).

This may secondarily increase absorption of iron (2). In addition to stimulating acid secretion, ethanol disrupts the mucosal barrier (3), and is an accepted cause of acute gastritis. This may be one of the mechanisms by which alcohol diminishes dietary intake. Alcohol may also impair gastric emptying (4).

Chronic ethanol administration first results in increased mean daily acid secretion and then gradually decreases it (5). The role of alcohol in the genesis of duodenal and gastric ulcer and chronic gastritis remains unsettled (6).

Alcohol has also been shown to be directly injurious to the small intestine (7). Acute administration of ethanol (1 g/kg) by mouth results in endoscopic and morphologic lesions in the duodenum (8). Previous failure to observe such lesions may have been due to their transient and patchy nature (9). Experimentally, such lesions are related to the concentration of ethanol used, with the greatest damage resulting from those solutions with the highest concentration of ethanol (10). Acute administration of ethanol may impair the absorption of many nutrients and experimentally results in alterations in mucosal enzymes (10–12).

Studies with oral and intravenous alcohol have revealed an inhibition of type I (impeding) waves in the jejunum and an increase in type III waves (propulsive waves) in the ileum (13). These changes have been proposed as one possible mechanism of the diarrhea observed in binge drinkers. Ingestion of ethanol has recently been demonstrated to result in release of secretin from the duodenum (14).

The effect of chronic ethanol consumption on intestinal function is complicated by the concomitant effects of nutrition. Indeed, malnutrition itself may lead to intestinal malabsorption (15, 16). Folate depletion, which is common in alcoholics, has been especially implicated in this regard (17–20). Impaired absorption of folate, thiamine, $B_{12}$, xylose, and fat has been described in alcoholics, with recovery after withdrawal from alcohol and institution of a nutritious diet (18, 21–24).

The absorption of water and electrolytes from the jejunum was studied in 10 alcoholics using a triple-lumen tube perfusion system (25). The mean rate of absorption of water in the alcoholic subjects (50.0 ± 2.3 ml/h) was significantly lower ($p < 0.001$) than the mean value in 14 healthy control subjects (205 ± 15.9 ml/h). Significant reduction in $Na^+$ and $Cl^-$ absorption was also demonstrated in the alcoholic subjects. These results indicate that alcoholics, after acute alcohol abuse, may have a functional impairment of water and electrolyte absorption from the jejunum. This may, in part, account for symptoms such as diarrhea, which may be present (25). However, generally the biochemical evidence of malabsorption correlates poorly with intestinal symptoms in the alcoholic (26).

Food intolerance, particularly of lactose, secondary to defective intestinal digestion could contribute to the production of these symptoms. Low lactase activity in adulthood exists in a majority of the world's population (27). Furthermore, location of lactase on the villus (28) makes it vulnerable to the corrosive effect of luminal toxins such as alcohol (10, 29). Indeed, disaccharidase activities often decrease with intestinal injury (30–32). To ascertain whether alcohol ingestion affects intestinal disaccharidase activities and influences the incidence of symptomatic lactose intolerance, lactase activity and lactose tolerance were studied in alcoholics and nonalcoholics of two human population groups with genetically determined low and high intestinal lactase levels, namely, blacks and whites (of northern European origin) (33). After an overnight fast, biopsies of the jejunum were obtained with a Quinton Multipurpose Suction Biopsy Tube positioned fluoroscopically at the level of the ligament of Treitz. When measured within 10 days of alcohol withdrawal, sucrase activity was decreased by 33% in the alcoholics. Lactase activity was less than 1 U/g in 100% of the black and 20% of the white alcoholics as compared to 50% of the black and none of the white controls. Lactase activity was virtually absent in 45% of the black alcoholics. A second jejunal biopsy following an additional 2 week period of alcohol abstinence exhibited significant secondary increases in the activities of both disaccharidases. Oral administration of lactose (1 g/kg body weight) resulted in significantly lower blood glucose concentration and higher incidence of adverse effects in alcoholics, mainly among the blacks.

The mechanism for the disaccharidase depression in alcoholics has not been fully elucidated. Since these effects were observed in alcoholics without nutritional deficiencies, the reduction in disaccharidase activity appears to be an effect of chronic alcohol ingestion per se. Ethanol administration to human volunteers for 3–6 days has been reported to inhibit glycolytic and gluconeogenic intestinal enzyme activities (34).

Similar depressions of intestinal disaccharidase as well as alkaline phosphatase activities have been produced in rats ingesting alcohol either acutely or chronically with nutritionally adequate diets (10). The dose of ethanol given to these rats resulted in ethanol concentrations within the intestinal lumen comparable to those found in human subjects after drinking (19). Evidence of gut injury and subsequent regeneration of intestinal epithelium has been found in rats fed diets containing ethanol (10), and in humans endoscoped after controlled alcohol administration (8). The concomitant improvement in disaccharidase activities and increase in mitotic activity after alcohol abstinence (33) are consistent with the possibility of regeneration. However, it is intriguing that the time required for the disaccharidase activities to improve was considerably longer than that expected for the epithelium to regenerate. This suggests that these effects of alcohol may reflect not merely villus cell desquamation, but also altered cell renewal or maturation. The low values of lactase activity in the jejunal biopsies of alcoholics were also accompanied by poor lactose absorption, as measured by the rise in blood glucose concentration after an oral load. This indicates that the alteration produced by alcohol was not restricted to the upper segment of the jejunum, but was sufficiently extended as to impair total lactose absorption. This effect was again more apparent in the black alcoholics. Lactose malabsorption was associated with increased incidence of colic, diarrhea, and a dumping-like syndrome severe enough to require medical attention. Thus, disaccharidase deficiency in alcoholics may be an indication of the damaging effect of alcohol on the intestinal epithelium, and may also lead to increased morbidity from primary lactase deficiency, a rather common disorder. As little as 3 g of lactose has been shown to produce symptoms in individuals with low intestinal lactase activities (35). Thus, milk intolerance may be unmasked or exaggerated in those populations where both alcoholism and genetically determined low lactase levels are common. In view of the likelihood of significant milk intolerance in alcoholics, the common practice of liberal milk supplementation for "nutritional restoration" or the treatment of gastritis or ulcer-associated symptoms should be reconsidered, particularly in ethnic groups (such as blacks) with preexisting low lactase activities.

The acute and chronic effects of alcohol on small intestinal function may be potentiated by concomitant alterations in pancreatic function, bile salts, and small intestinal flora. However, in patients with cirrhosis, steatorrhea (fecal fat greater than 30 g/24 hours on a 100 g fat/day diet) is relatively uncommon and in one series was present in only 9% of cases (36). Portal hypertension has also been postulated as a cause of malabsorption (37). Finally, specific therapeutic interventions, such as neomycin, may by themselves cause malabsorption (38). Chronic pancreatitis may lead to pancreatic insufficiency in the alcoholic and may contribute to steatorrhea and malabsorption. Acute pancreatitis may result in diminished dietary intake and severe fluid and electrolyte disturbances. Both acute and chronic pancreatitis may cause alterations in glucose tolerance.

Acute and chronic alcohol administration as well as alcoholic liver disease have each been noted to alter bile salt metabolism. Acutely, administration of ethanol intravenously or into the jejunum decreases intraluminal bile salts (39). Chronic ethanol feeding in the rat prolongs the half excretion time of cholic and chenodeoxycholic acid, increases the pool size slightly, and decreases daily excretion (40).

## ALCOHOL, MALNUTRITION, AND THE PATHOGENESIS OF ALCOHOLIC LIVER INJURY

The question of the respective roles of alcohol and malnutrition in the pathogenesis of liver disease seen in the alcoholic (fatty liver, alcoholic hepatitis, and cirrhosis) is very significant both for the prevention and for the treatment of the disease. The resolution of this question has been exceedingly difficult for several reasons: the unreliability of alcoholic populations, the variability of disease expression, the difficulty of accurate nutritional evaluation, and the long time course of pathogenesis.

Malnutrition has been proposed as the predominant factor producing liver injury for several reasons. Each gram of ethanol provides 7.1 calories, which means that 20 ounces (or 586 ml) of 86 proof (43% v/v) beverage represents about 1500 calories or one-half to two-thirds of the normal daily caloric requirement. Therefore, the alcoholic has a much reduced demand for food to fulfill his caloric needs. Since alcoholic beverages do not contain significant amounts of protein, vitamins, and minerals, the intake of these nutrients may become borderline or insufficient. Economic factors may also reduce the consumption of nutrient-rich food by the alcoholic. In addition to acting as "empty" or "naked" calories, alcohol can result in malnutrition by interfering with the normal processes of food digestion and absorption (26).

For all these reasons, deficiency diseases readily develop in the alcoholic. In rodents, severely deficient diets result in liver damage even in the absence of alcohol. Extrapolation from these animal results to man led to the belief that in alcoholics, the liver disease is due not to ethanol but solely to the nutritional deficiencies, and that given an adequate diet alcohol is merely acting by its caloric contribution and that it is not more toxic than a similar caloric load derived from fats or starches (41). This opinion prevailed, despite some statistical evidence gathered both in France (42) and in Germany (43), which indicated that the incidence of liver disease correlated with the amount of alcohol consumed rather than with deficiencies in the diet. A major challenge to the concept of the exclusively nutritional origin of alcoholic liver disease arose from an improvement of the method of feeding alcohol to experimental animals. Indeed, when the conventional alcohol feeding procedure is used, namely, when ethanol is given as part of the drinking water, rats usually refuse to take a sufficient amount of ethanol to develop liver injury, if the diet is adequate. This aversion of rats to ethanol was counteracted by the introduction of the new technique of feeding of ethanol as part of a nutritionally adequate totally liquid diet (44–46). With this procedure, ethanol intake was sufficient to produce a fatty liver despite an adequate diet. This technique has been widely adopted for the study of the pathogenesis of the fatty liver in the rat. In addition to the fatty liver, ethanol dependence developed in these rats, as indicated by typical withdrawal seizures after cessation of alcohol intake (47).

Having established an etiologic role for ethanol in the pathogenesis of the experimental fatty liver, the question of its importance for the development of human pathology remained. To determine whether ingestion of alcohol, in amounts comparable to those consumed by chronic alcoholics, is capable of injuring the liver even in the absence of dietary deficiencies, volunteers (with or without a history of alcoholism) were given a variety of nondeficient diets under metabolic ward conditions, with ethanol either as a supplement to the diet or as an isocaloric substitution for carbohydrates (44, 45, 48). In all these individuals, ethanol administration resulted in the development of fatty liver, which was evident both on morphologic examination and by direct measurement of the lipid content of the liver biopsies which revealed an increase in triglyceride concentration up to fifteenfold.

The etiologic role of alcohol per se (in the absence of dietary deficiency) in the pathogenesis of alcoholic liver injury has now been extended from the fatty liver to the full spectrum of liver disease, including cirrhosis. This was achieved by using an experimental model developed in the baboon (49); in these experimental animals, the sequential development

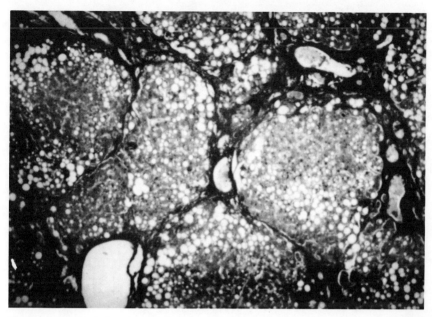

**Figure 1.**   Cirrhosis in a baboon fed alcohol for four years. Fat is regularly distributed through liver nodules surrounded by connective septa. Chromotropeaniline blue (×42) (49).

of all the liver lesions seen in the alcoholic was reproduced: to date in 24 baboons fed ethanol all developed fatty liver, five progressed to mild hepatitis, and nine had cirrhosis, complete in seven (Figure 1), and incomplete in two. Maintenance of a nutritionally adequate regimen despite the intake of inebriating amounts of ethanol (50% of total calories) was achieved by incorporating the ethanol into a totally liquid diet. On ethanol withdrawal, signs of physical dependence, such as seizures and tremors, developed. Ultrastructural changes of the mitochondria and the endoplasmic reticulum were already present at the fatty liver stage, and persisted throughout the cirrhosis. The lesions were similar to those observed in alcoholics and differed from the alterations produced by choline and protein deficiencies. At the fatty liver stage, some "adaptive" increases in the activity of microsomal enzymes (aniline hydroxylase and microsomal ethanol-oxidizing system, MEOS) were observed, but these tended to disappear with the development of hepatitis and cirrhosis. Fat accumulation was also much more pronounced in the animals with hepatitis, as compared to those with simple fatty liver (an eighteenfold, compared to a threefold to fourfold, increase in liver triglycerides). The

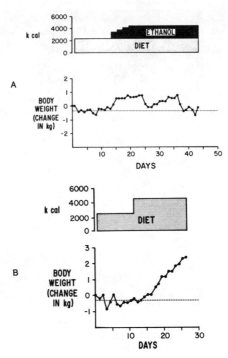

**Figure 2.** Effect on body weight of the addition of 2000 kcal/day as ethanol (A) or as chocolate (B) to the diet of the same subject. The dotted line represents the mean change during the control period (52).

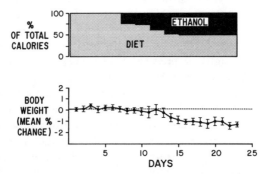

**Figure 3.** Body weight changes after isocaloric substitution of ethanol (50% of total calories) for carbohydrate in 11 subjects (means ± standard errors). The dotted line represents the mean change in weight in control period (52).

160

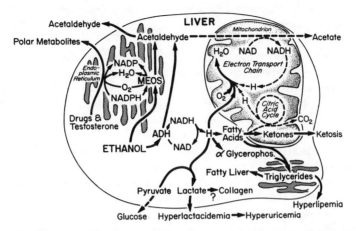

**Figure 4.** Oxidation of ethanol in the hepatocyte and its link to fatty liver, hyperlipemia, hyperuricemia, hyperlactacidemia, ketosis, hypoglycemia, and drug and acetaldehyde metabolism. NAD denotes nicotinamide adenine dinucleotide, NADH reduced NAD, NADP nicotinamide adenine dinucleotide phosphate, NADPH reduced NADP, MEOS the microsomal ethanol-oxidizing system, and ADH alcohol dehydrogenase. The broken lines indicate pathways that are depressed by ethanol (64).

demonstration that these lesions can develop despite an adequate diet indicates that in addition to correction of the nutritional status, control of alcohol intake is mandatory for the management of patients with alcoholic liver injury, and that ethanol per se must be considered a direct etiologic agent in the pathogenesis of alcoholic liver injury, independent of dietary factors (50). However, this does not preclude the possibility that dietary factors may contribute to and potentiate the alcohol effect, which has previously been shown to be the case in rats (51). No similar studies are available for man.

## THE NUTRITIONAL VALUE OF ALCOHOLIC BEVERAGES

Ethanol liberates 7.1 kcal/g when combusted, but does not provide equivalent caloric food value when compared to carbohydrate. Gain in body weight is significantly lower with ethanol than with isocaloric amounts of carbohydrate (52) (Figure 2), and isocaloric substitution of ethanol for carbohydrate as 50% of total calories in a balanced diet results in a decline in body weight (52) (Figure 3). One interpretation of this lack of weight gain with ethanol compared to other sources of dietary calories is the possibility that chronic alcohol intake increases the energy requirements of the body. If this were the case, it should be reflected in a higher rate of oxygen consumption. It was indeed found in rats fed alcohol as part of their totally liquid diet that oxygen consumption was slightly but significantly higher than that of animals pair-fed the isocaloric diet containing carbohydrates instead of ethanol (53).

Among the many mechanisms that could be postulated to account for an inefficient use of ethanol calories, one involves the energy wastage secondary to an induction of liver microsomal pathways and increased ethanol oxidation at this accessory site.

Efficient utilization of the calories of ethanol would be anticipated from a consideration of its major metabolic pathway, which involves the hepatic cytosolic enzyme alcohol dehydrogenase (ADH) (Figure 4).

From an energy point of view, this process appears to be an economical one because the associated production of NADH supplies the electron transport chain with hydrogen equivalents, yielding high-energy phosphate bonds. In addition to the ADH pathway, ethanol is also metabolized via a hepatic miscrosomal ethanol-oxidizing system (MEOS) (54). The exact quantitative significance of the enzyme system in vivo remains uncertain, but studies indicate that it could normally involve 20–25% of the oxidation of ethanol (55) and much more after chronic ethanol consumption, particularly at high ethanol concentrations (56). The potential importance of this in the body's caloric balance lies in the fact that in contrast to the ADH pathway, MEOS results in the loss of chemical energy from both the substrate and the cofactor (NADPH), without any known effective coupling to ATP synthesis (Figure 4). Presumably, the chemical energy is dissipated as heat. The latter, insofar as it exceeds the body's thermoregulatory needs, represents an inefficient use of ingested calories. In support of this theory is the recent observation of increased body temperature after alcohol (61). It is of interest that similar considerations apply to the oxidation of other drugs and endogenous substrates (such as steroids) by hepatic microsomal drug-metabolizing enzymes. These oxidations have the general formula:

$$RH + NADPH + H^+ + O_2 \rightarrow ROH + NADP^+ + H_2O$$

The proposed hypothesis (53) is that the inefficiency of microsomal drug-metabolizing enzymes could be of quantitative significance in the energy balance of the body during the repeated intake of drugs, especially ethanol. The hypothesis is in keeping with other animal studies in which metabolic rates were increased by the administration of ethanol and barbiturates in doses known to induce hepatic microsomal enzymes. Thus, pretreatment with barbiturates enhanced oxygen consumption in rats tested under various conditions: in the absence of drugs, during hexobarbital anesthesia, and after the administration of aminopyrine (57).

There are, of course, many metabolic pathways in the body that are not effectively linked to ATP synthesis. These pathways contribute to the net wastage of calories to give a less than optimal overall efficiency of the body. In this respect, the microsomal drug-metabolizing enzyme system is unique in its extraordinary versatility and in its ability to be induced by a wide variety of agents.

Another major theory is that the hypermetabolic state produced by ethanol is caused by an increased utilization of ATP by the $Na^+$-$K^+$-activated ATPase after chronic ethanol feeding. Israel and co-workers (58) reported that in liver slices, ouabain, an inhibitor of the $Na^+$-$K^+$-activated ATPase, can completely block the extra ethanol metabolism elicited by chronic ethanol treatment. Dinitrophenol increased the rate of ethanol metabolism in the livers of the treated animals only in the presence of ouabain.

The theory that increased utilization of ATP by the $Na^+$-$K^+$-activated ATPase (and the lowering of the phosphorylation potential that results) is responsible for the metabolic adaptation that occurs in rats after chronic ethanol treatment, and that a situation develops that is very similar to that found after administration of thyroid hormones or epinephrine, is intriguing. Certainly, the influence of ethanol consumption on hormonal actions deserves further investigation. To date, there have been few studies performed to confirm these observations.

Under the conditions used by Israel and co-workers (58), ethanol consumption did not result in liver changes comparable to those seen in human alcoholic liver injury; for instance, no fatty liver was observed. Under conditions that mimic the clinical situation with development of fatty liver, chronic ethanol consumption was not found to be associated with increased ATPase activity (59), and the increase in the rates of ethanol metabolism after chronic ethanol consumption could not be abolished by ouabain (60), which indicates that the theory of enhanced ATPase activity may not be applicable to the situation that normally prevails after chronic alcohol consumption.

In summary, malnutrition is common among alcoholics because alcohol, high in caloric value, displaces other foods in the diet. Each gram of ethanol provides 7.1 calories. Therefore the alcoholic has a reduced demand for food to fulfill his caloric needs. Moreover, the calories provided by alcohol do not fully "count," at least at relatively high levels of intake, especially among alcoholics. One of the pathways of ethanol metabolism (MEOS) is wasteful because it is not associated with formation of high-energy phosphate bonds; therefore, heat is produced without conservation of chemical energy. Furthermore, alcoholic beverages contain few, if any, vitamins, minerals, protein, or other nutrients. The alcoholic's intake of foods containing these nutrients may readily become insufficient.

Chronic alcohol consumption can also result in malnutrition by interfering with normal food digestion and absorption. Alcohol exerts a direct effect on the gut and pancreas. At high concentrations, it causes erosions of the gastrointestinal mucosa. Even in the absence of these lesions, alcohol abuse reduces intestinal enzymes (e.g., lactase). Alcohol may also impair absorption of various essential nutrients, including vitamins $B_1$ and $B_{12}$. A number of alcoholics also have a history of poor protein intake which may result in protein depletion. However, it is somewhat difficult to differentiate protein deficiency from decreased protein production as a result of liver disease. Protein repletion must, therefore, be carried out cautiously in the alcoholic, since protein overload in those with severe liver disease may be harmful. Alcohol is also a direct cause of alcoholic liver disease. Indeed, in baboons the entire spectrum of alcoholic liver disease can be produced by administration of ethanol despite nutritionally adequate diets and the absence of abnormal intestinal losses of nutrients. Fatty liver develops when alcohol replaces fat as the preferred energy source for the liver. Combustion of fat ceases and lipid accumulates in the liver. Although in absolute amounts, lipoprotein secretion is enhanced (leading to hyperlipemia), relative to the availability of fat, it is insufficient to prevent steatosis. There is proliferation of the smooth membranes of the endoplasmic reticulum, with increased activity of various microsomal drug metabolizing and ethanol oxidizing enzymes. There is swelling of the mitochondria, with reduced oxidation of fat (again promoting steatosis) and of acetaldehyde, the product of ethanol oxidation in the liver. Elevated acetaldehyde levels enhance the toxicity of ethanol. Progression of the liver damage is associated with a decrease in serum lipids, exaggeration of steatosis, and deposition of fibrous tissue (initially in the centrolobular zones), leading to development of cirrhosis despite an adequate diet. Therefore, alcoholics should not be led to believe that mere correction or prevention of nutritional inadequacies will fully protect against liver damage, though associated deficiencies (particularly of folate and thiamine) mandate treatment.

## THE NUTRITIONAL STATUS OF THE ALCOHOLIC

Alcoholism remains one of the few causes of florid nutritional deficiencies in our society. However, the stereotype of the malnourished alcoholic is probably unfounded as it applies to the millions of alcoholics in the

United States. The spread of alcoholism to various socioeconomic classes, the greater availability and enrichment of foods, and the investigation of broader populations of alcoholics have led to a modification of this view. Indeed, moderate alcohol consumption was found to have little impact on nutritional status (62) and no significant differences have been found among alcoholics and nonalcoholics matched for socioeconomic and health history (63). Nevertheless, alcohol may interact with nutrition at many levels to produce marginal if not clinically overt deficiencies. These interactions are summarized in Table 1. The clinical significance of such nutritional deficiencies by themselves or in conjunction with alcohol with regard to organ damage in the alcoholic remains an interesting area for further exploration. Moreover, alcohol abuse is associated with several metabolic disorders such as hyperlipemia, hyperuricemia, and ketoacidosis (Figure 3). Their impact through interaction with nutritionally conditioned abnormalities still deserves assessment in our general population.

# REFERENCES

1. W. Y. Chey, *Digestion*, **7**, 239 (1972).
2. R. W. Charlton, P. Jacobs, H. Seftel, and T. H. Bothwell, *Brit. Med. J.*, **2**, 1427 (1964).
3. H. W. Davenport, *Gastroenterology*, **56**, 439 (1969).
4. J. J. Barboriak and R. C. Meade, *Am. J. Clin. Nutr.*, **23**, 1151 (1970).
5. W. Y. Chey, S. Kosay, and S. H. Lorber, *Dig. Dis.*, **17**, 153 (1972).
6. S. H. Lorber, V. P. Dinoso, and W. Y. Chey, in B. Kissin and H. Begleiter, Eds., *Biology of Alcoholism*, Plenum Press, New York, 1974, p. 339.
7. E. Rubin, B. Rybak, J. Lindenbaum, C. D. Gerson, G. Walker, and C. S. Lieber, *Gastroenterology*, **63**, 801 (1972).
8. E. B. Gottfried, M. A. Korsten, and C. S. Lieber, *Am. J. Gastroenterology*, in press (1979).
9. R. C. Pirola, T. D. Bolin, and A. E. Davis, *Am. J. Dig. Dis.*, **14**, 239 (1969).
10. E. Baraona, R. C. Pirola, and C. S. Lieber, *Gastroenterology*, **66**, 226 (1974).
11. Y. Israel, J. E. Valenzuela, I. Salazar, and G. Ugarte, *J. Nutr.*, **98**, 222 (1969).
12. R. W. Hillman, in B. Kissin and H. Begleiter, Eds., *Biology of Alcoholism*, Plenum Press, New York, 1974, p. 513.
13. E. A. Robles, E. Mezey, C. H. Halsted, and M. M. Schuster, *Johns Hopkins Med. J.*, **135**, 17 (1974).
14. E. Straus, E. J. Croach, and R. S. Yalow, *New Engl. J. Med.*, **293**, 1301 (1975).
15. W. P. T. James, *Lancet*, **1**, 333 (1968).
16. L. G. Mayoral, K. Tripahty, F. T. Garcia, S. Klahr, O. Bolanos, and J. Ghitis, *Am. J. Clin. Nutr.*, **20**, 866 (1967).

17. S. J. Winawer, L. W. Sullivan, V. Herbert, and N. Zamcheck, *New Engl. J. Med.,* **272,** 892 (1965).

18. C. H. Halsted, E. A. Robles, and E. Mezey, *New Engl. J. Med.,* **285,** 701 (1971).

19. C. H. Halsted, E. A. Robles, and E. Mezey, *Gastroenterology,* **64,** 526 (1973).

20. J. A. Hermos, W. H. Adams, Y. K. Lui, L. W. Sullivan, and J. S. Trier, *Ann. Intern. Med.,* **76,** 957 (1972).

21. J. Lindenbaum and C. S. Lieber, in M. K. Roach, W. M. McIsaac, and P. J. Creaven, Eds., *Proceedings of the Symposium on Biological Aspects of Alcohol,* Vol. 3, University of Texas Press, Austin, 1971, p. 27.

22. P. A. Tomasula, R. M. H. Kater, and F. L. Iber, *Am. J. Clin. Nutr.,* **21,** 1340 (1968).

23. G. M. Roggin, F. L. Iber, R. M. H. Kater, and F. Tobon, *Johns Hopkins Med. J.,* **125,** 321 (1969).

24. E. Mezey, E. Jow, R. W. Slavin, and F. Tobon, *Gastroenterology,* **59,** 657 (1970).

25. N. Krasner, K. M. Cochran, R. I. Russell, H. A. Carmichael, and G. G. Thompson, *Gut,* **17,** 245 (1976).

26. J. Lindenbaum and C. S. Lieber, *Ann. N.Y. Acad. Sci.,* **252,** 228 (1975).

27. T. M. Bayless, D. M. Paige, and G. D. Ferry, *Gastroenterology,* **60,** 605 (1971).

28. C. Nordstrom, A. Dahlqvist, and L. Josefsson, *J. Histochem. Cytochem.,* **15,** 713 (1968).

29. E. Baraona, R. C. Pirola, and C. S. Lieber, *Biochim. Biophys. Acta,* **338,** 19 (1975).

30. J. J. Herbst, R. Hurwitz, P. Sunshine, and N. Kretchmer, *J. Clin. Invest.,* **49,** 530 (1970).

31. P. Berchtold, A. Dahlqvist, A. Gustafson, and N.-G. Asp, *Scand. J. Gastroenterology,* **6,** 751 (1971).

32. R. A. Giannella, W. R. Routh, and P. P. Toskes, *Gastroenterology,* **67,** 965 (1971).

33. W. Perlow, E. Baraona and C. S. Lieber, *Gastroenterology,* **72,** 680 (1977).

34. H. L. Greene, F. B. Stifel, R. H. Herman, Y. F. Herman, and N. S. Rosensweig, *Gastroenterology,* **67,** 434 (1974).

35. M. S. Bedine and T. M. Bayless, *Gastroenterology,* **65,** 735 (1973).

36. W. G. Linscheer, *Am. J. Clin. Nutr.,* **23,** 488 (1970).

37. M. S. Losowsky and B. E. Walker, *Gastroenterology,* **56,** 589 (1969).

38. W. W. Faloon, *Am. J. Clin. Nutr.,* **23,** 645 (1970).

39. G. A. Marin, N. L. Ward, and R. Fischer, *Dig. Dis.,* **18,** 825 (1973).

40. A. F. Lefevre, L. M. DeCarli, and C. S. Lieber, *J. Lipid Res.,* **13,** 48 (1972).

41. C. H. Best, W. S. Hartroft, C. C. Lucas and J. H. Ridout, *Brit. Med. J.,* **2,** 1001 (1949).

42. G. Pequignot, *Muchen. Med. Wschr.,* **103,** 1464 (1962).

43. W. K. Lelbach, *Acta Hepatosplen.,* **14,** 9 (1967).

44. C. S. Lieber, D. P. Jones, J. Mendelson and L. M. DeCarli, *Trans. Assn. Amer. Physicians,* **76,** 289 (1963).

45. C. S. Lieber, D. P. Jones and L. M. DeCarli, *J. Clin. Invest,* **44,** 1009 (1965).

46. L. M. DeCarli and C. S. Lieber, *J. Nutr.,* **91,** 331 (1967).

47. C. S. Lieber and L. M. DeCarli, *Res. Commun. Chem. Path. Pharmacol.,* **6,** 983 (1973).

48. C. S. Lieber and E. Rubin, *Am. J. Med.,* **44,** 200 (1968).

49. C. S. Lieber and L. M. DeCarli, *J. Med. Primatology,* **3,** 153 (1974).

50. C. S. Lieber, L. M. DeCarli and E. Rubin, *Proc. Nat. Acad. Sci.,* **72,** 437 (1975).

51. C. S. Lieber, N. Spritz and L. M. DeCarli, *J. Lipid Res.,* **10,** 283 (1969).

52. R. C. Pirola and C. S. Lieber, *Pharmacol.,* **7,** 185 (1972).

53. R. C. Pirola and C. S. Lieber, *Am. J. Clin. Nutr.,* **29,** 90 (1976).

54. C. S. Lieber and L. M. DeCarli, *J. Biol. Chem.,* **245,** 2505 (1970).

55. C. S. Lieber and L. M. DeCarli, *J. Pharmacol. Exp. Ther.,* **181,** 278 (1972).

56. S. Matsuzaki, R. Teschke, K. Ohnishi, and C. S. Lieber, in M. M. Fisher and J. G. Rankin, Eds., *Alcohol and the Liver,* Plenum Press, New York, Vol. 3, 1977, p. 119.

57. R. C. Pirola and C. S. Lieber, *J. Nutr.,* **105,** 1544 (1975).

58. Y. Israel, L. Videla, V. Fernandes-Videal, and J. Bernstein, *J. Pharmacol. Exp. Ther.,* **192,** 565 (1975).

59. E. R. Gordon, *Alcoholism: Clin. Exper. Res.,* **1,** 21 (1977).

60. A. I. Cederbaum, E. Dicker, H. Gang, C. S. Lieber, and E. Rubin, *Fed. Proc.,* **35,** 1709 (1976).

61. E. A. Hosein and B. Bexton, *Biochem. Pharmacol.,* **24,** 1859 (1975).

62. H. T. Bebb, H. B. Houser, J. C. Witschi, A. S. Littell, and R. K. Fuller, *Am. J. Clin. Nutr.,* **24,** 1042 (1971).

63. W. W. Westerfeld and M. P. Schulman, *J. A. M. A.,* **170,** 197 (1959).

64. C. S. Lieber, *New Engl. J. Med.,* **298,** 888 (1978).

# 11

# Gastrointestinal Surgery as it Affects Nutrition

ELLIOT WESER, M.D.

University of Texas Medical School, San Antonio, Texas

Various surgical procedures on the gastrointestinal tract may have profound effects on patient nutrition. These effects usually result either from a significant reduction in food intake or from malabsorption as a complication of the surgical procedure. Reduced food intake is seen particularly after gastric surgery. The usual causes for this may be distention, gastritis in the gastric remnant, dumping syndrome with diarrhea, the occurrence of late postprandial hypoglycemia (usually 1 to 2 hours after meals), or finally, afferent loop obstruction. The effect of each of these conditions, if not treated, will be a reduction of food intake to avoid the occurrence of symptoms. Actually, reduced caloric intake is the major reason for weight loss in patients subsequent to a partial gastrectomy. Whereas the dumping syndrome and late postprandial hypoglycemia may be effectively treated by medical dietary methods, correction of a distended gastric remnant due to either a stenosed jejunostomy stoma or an obstruction of the afferent loop often requires surgical revision of the initial operation.

Gastrointestinal surgery may also significantly affect the nutrition of the patient by producing malabsorption. Malabsorption may be either a direct consequence of surgery or a developing complication. Postgastrectomy malabsorption is a well-defined entity in some patients following a partial gastric resection. The patient with a partial gastrectomy who has a progressive downhill course with significant diarrhea and weight loss must be evaluated for the existence of malabsorption. Often these pa-

**169**

tients also do not ingest adequate calories because of their debility and desire to reduce symptoms. Evaluation for malabsorption is therefore important to approach their management properly. The proximal small intestine, particularly the duodenum, is the site of maximal transport of both iron and calcium, although the remaining part of the small bowel also absorbs these ions. A Billroth type 2 gastrectomy with bypass of the duodenum may result in impaired iron and calcium absorption and hence can lead to a deficiency of these minerals. Iron loss from gastritis in the gastric remnant will also contribute to iron deficiency. Calcium deficiency may be a particular problem in postmenopausal women who have undergone this surgical procedure. Similarly, duodenal bypass of the proximal intestine in this operation may result in inadequate absorption of dietary folates and thus lead to a folic acid deficiency. Again, reduced intake of folate may also contribute. The proper absorption of dietary sources of vitamin $B_{12}$ requires intrinsic factor, which is depleted when the stomach is removed. In man, intrinsic factor is thought to be produced in parietal cells. With removal of significant portions of the parietal cell portion of the stomach, and with gastric atrophy occurring in the remnant of the stomach (because of chronic gastritis), vitamin $B_{12}$ absorption over several years may be impaired sufficiently that the patient develops a $B_{12}$ deficiency. Another malabsorptive problem seen after gastrectomy is the malabsorption of lactose due to the unmasking of a previously existing lactase deficit. In the absence of a stomach, any lactose that is ingested may rapidly enter the proximal intestine, and the load that presents itself to the intestine at any one time is more than prior to the surgery, so that symptoms of lactose intolerance become apparent. Fat malabsorption is most important nutritionally after gastrectomy and may occur for several reasons. Afferent loop stasis after a Billroth type 2 operation may permit the overgrowth of bacteria in the afferent loop and the proximal intestine. The increased bacteria deconjugate bile salts and result in faulty fat micelle formation, with reduced absorption of fat. The resulting steatorrhea may also be associated with malabsorption of vitamin D and impaired absorption of dietary calcium. If this condition is untreated, metabolic bone disease may develop, particularly in postmenopausal women. Another cause of fat malabsorption after a Billroth type 2 gastrectomy may be relative pancreatic enzyme deficinecy. Several factors may cause this. A faulty secretogogue response to food entering the efferent limb, with inadequate enzyme mixing and maldigestion of ingested food is one. If a patient has a significant amount of weight loss and cachexia following a gastric procedure, primary pancreatic atrophy can occur and contribute to decreased enzyme secretion. Finally, after a gastrectomy the small bowel may be subjected to excessively large, undiluted doses of the wheat protein, gluten, and this may unmask a previously existing celiac sprue condition. There are numerous cases reported in which classic celiac sprue disease was uncovered subsequent to a gastrectomy.

Gastrointestinal surgery may also cause malabsorption by creating blind loop syndromes, in addition to the malabsorption associated with gastrectomy and afferent loop stasis. For example, fistulae, partial bowel obstruction, and atonic loops of bowel may occur subsequent to surgery. These conditions may be associated with overgrowth of bacteria in the small bowel and can result in both steatorrhea and impaired vitamin $B_{12}$ absorption. The bacteria compete for the vitamin $B_{12}$, bind it, and reduce its availability for intestinal transport.

Obviously, surgical procedures involving a complete pancreatectomy will result in exocrine (and endocrine) enzyme deficiency and maldigestion-malabsorption.

Perhaps the most common cause of malabsorption after gastrointestinal surgery involves extensive small bowel resection, bypass, or the creation of large enteric fistulae. The degree of malabsorption following small bowel resection depends on the extent and site of the resection, the presence of the ileocecal valve, the condition of remaining bowel, liver, and pancreas, and finally, the degree to which the remaining intestine undergoes adaptation in response to the shortened state. There are numerous causes of short bowel, including abdominal trauma, mesenteric thrombosis, regional enteritis, small bowel obstruction, such as volvulus, carcinoma, and lymphoma of the small bowel, radiation enteropathy, and the jejunoileal bypass. Malabsorption after small bowel resection obviously depends on the extent and the specific site of intestine removed. For example, most nutrients are absorbed from the proximal half to two-thirds of the small intestine. This includes fat, carbohydrates, proteins, and most of the vitamins. The ileum, however, is specifically adapted to actively transport vitamin $B_{12}$ and reabsorb conjugated bile acids in an ileohepatic circulation. Metabolites of vitamin D may also be absorbed via an ileohepatic circulation as an important mechanism for the conservation of 25-OH vitamin D. Extensive resections of the small bowel will obviously reduce the absorbable length of intestine and impair transport of many nutrients. However, a resection involving just the ileum can result in loss of bile salts into the colon, producing a secretory diarrhea as a result of inhibition of sodium and water transport in the colon. Ultimately this may result in a deficiency of bile salt in the proximal intestine, causing chronic steatorrhea. Thus, even limited resections of the ileum may result in malabsorption of bile acids, diarrhea, steatorrhea, and vitamin $B_{12}$ malabsorption. Other effects of small bowel resection are a sequel to the steatorrhea, and involve the malabsorption of calcium and magnesium and the fat-soluble vitamins A, D, and K. A complication appreciated in relatively recent years has been the excessive excretion of oxalate in the urine in patients who have small bowel resection or other chronic steatorrheic states. Under normal circumstances dietary oxalate binds with dietary and intraluminal calcium to form calcium oxalate, which is insoluble and precipitates out. Therefore the oxalate is not available for absorption. In the presence of steatorrhea, unabsorbed fatty acids bind dietary calcium and this renders the oxalate in the diet more soluble, and hence absorbable. The site of absorption of dietary oxalate has been shown to be in the colon. Over several years there is an increased frequency of formation of oxalate stones. Patients who have a colectomy in addition to a small intestinal resection do not develop hyperoxaluria and are at no greater risk to develop oxalate stones. The ileocecal valve may be an important factor in determining whether patients develop diarrhea after an ileectomy. Most ileectomies involve the ileocecal junction and in the absence of this area diarrhea is usually more severe. A shortened bowel may also permit bacteria in the colon to colonize the remaining small intestine, implicating a blind loop syndrome as another factor in the malabsorption that occurs after bowel resection.

It is apparent that the condition of remaining small intestine after a bowel resection as well as the state of liver and pancreatic function may contribute to the degree of malabsorption.

Finally, the extent to which the remaining intestine undergoes adaptation is an important factor in how a patient fares subsequent to extensive small bowel removal. It has long been appreciated that with time intestinal function improves after a small bowel resection. There is a reduction in steatorrhea and fecal nitrogen and increased segmental glucose, sodium, calcium, and water absorption per centimeter of remaining gut. Absorption of vitamin $B_{12}$ also increases with time. These events are thought to be associated with hyperplasia of the mucosa in the remaining intestine. It is of interest that this hyperplasia takes place in man and experimental animals only if nutrients are provided intraluminally either by oral ingestion or by instillation of nutrients into the bowel. Animals and man maintained on total parenteral nutrition and in positive caloric balance do not undergo this intestinal mucosal hyperplasia. Factors responsible for this phenomenon may be the direct transport of nutrients through the mucosa, stimulation of mucosal growth by bile and pancreatic secretions, trophic effects of enteric hormones, or neurovascular changes subsequent to small bowel resection.

It is apparent, therefore, that gastrointestinal surgery can influence human nutrition in a variety of ways. Reduced food intake may be an important consequence of some gastric procedures. Gastrointestinal surgery may also produce malabsorption, particularly when extensive resection of the small bowel is performed. Bacterial overgrowth in the small bowel, creating a blind loop syndrome, may occur as a singular event or may complicate a short bowel condition. Understanding the reasons for both reduced food intake and malabsorption after bowel surgery permits us to approach therapy rationally.

# 12

---

# Current Status of Surgery
# for Morbid Obesity

DAVID H. ALPERS, M.D., AND
JOHN D. HALVERSON, M.D.

Washington University School of Medicine, St. Louis, Missouri

Surgery for obesity in recent years has consisted mainly of two procedures: jejunoileal bypass and gastroplasty, or gastric bypass. The choice
of patients for these operations is based on the relationship between
obesity and increased mortality. When the body mass index (wt/ht$^2$)
exceeds 40, the equivalent of 40% overweight, the relative excess mortality approaches twice that for persons of normal weight (1). This body
mass index corresponds to a weight of 115–140 kg. However, less than
1% of the population exceeds 120 kg and less than 0.1% exceeds 140 kg.
No studies have been performed directly on this special group of patients
to determine their mortality or rate of illnesses such as hypertension.
Such studies are important if long-term benefits of operative intervention are to be assessed. Nevertheless, most patients selected for bypass
operations are in this group, since patients more than 100 lbs over standard for height, sex, and age are selected (2). In addition, these patients
must have failed at other forms of therapy. This failure is judged dif-
ferently by physicians. Since most patients have shown the ability to lose
weight by dietary restriction for a short period of time, what constitutes
"failure"? In practice it is the patient who determines this failure by
his presentation to a physician who will perform the operation. The patients to be selected must have no serious underlying disease except those
related to obesity. Finally, they must be psychiatrically and socially
stable. This requirement is difficult to evaluate. What is normal, when a

**175**

### Table 1    Complications of Gastric Bypass[a]

|  | % |
|---|---|
| Complications of operation | 25 |
| Wound infection | 4–13 |
| Chronic vomiting | 2–10 |
| Reflux esophagitis | 3 |
| Marginal ulcer | <2 |
| Dumping syndrome | <2 |
| Splenectomy | 2–3 |
| Death | 1–2 |

[a] These figures represent data from 2–3 year follow-ups from three separate series (Mason and co-workers (7), Hermrich and co-workers (8), and unpublished series of 173 patients from St. Louis).

significant percentage of the ambulatory population has emotional disorders (3)? Moreover, many obese patients eat compulsively, and this compulsive behavior affects their response to the operation. Clearly, these important issues need to be addressed but cannot be answered at the present time.

The short-term benefits of jejunoileal bypass include weight loss in all, lowering of blood pressure in hypertensive patients, and lowering of cholesterol and total lipids (4). Potential but undocumented long-term benefits include changes in mortality, and improved lifestyle. Some studies have claimed improvement in lifestyle (5) and emotional states (6), but these studies are somewhat flawed by the facts that not all patients in the series were examined before and after surgery, and that the self-answered questionnaires used in one study (5) would tend to give favorable results. It is always tempting for a patient to regard a major operation as worthwhile. In summary, the documented benefits of jejunoileal bypass surgery are largely cosmetic (weight loss), and perhaps more significant, so far, gastric bypass clearly accounts for a similar degree of weight loss (7, 8). Other benefits are undocumented at the present writing. However, our recent findings (see below) suggest that even weight loss may not be permanent after jejunoileal bypass.

The initial enthusiasm for jejunoileal bypass has been tempered by a growing list of complications. Jejunocolostomy is no longer performed and will not be further mentioned. Most of the material discussed will deal with complications of jejunoileal bypass, but the side effects of gastric bypass will also be covered briefly.

## Table 2  Late Complications of Jejunoileal Bypass[a]

| Complication | Incidence (%) | Treatment |
|---|---|---|
| Diarrhea | 13–98 | Low fat diet, opiates |
| Hypokalemia | 23–42 | K citrate 15–60 mEq/day |
| Hypocalcemia | 9–21 | $CaCO_3$ 1–2 g/day |
| Hypomagnesemia | (22) | Mg gluconate 1–3 g/day |
| Malnutrition/weakness | (14) | TPN, reversal |
| Nephrolithiasis | 7–13 | Low oxalate diet, $CaCO_3$ |
| Polyarthritis/arthralgias | 6/19 | Anti-inflammatory drugs |
| Biliary calculi | 7–10 | Cholecystectomy |
| Psychiatric illness | 7–9 | ? |
| Ventral hernia | 3–28 | Surgical repair |
| Anemia | 6–11 | Folic acid, $B_{12}$, iron |
| Progressive liver disease | | |
|   Irreversible fibrosis or | | |
|     cirrhosis | 4–8 | TPN, reversal |
|   Reversible fat, fibrosis, | | |
|     inflammation | 6–20 | |
|   Death | 1–2 | |
| Vitamin deficiency | | |
|   (blood levels) | | |
|   Folic acid | (45) Preop (81) | Folate 1 mg/day |
|   Vitamin D | (42) Osteopenia (8) | 50,000 IU/day vitamin D |
| | | three times per week |
|   Vitamin A | (42) | 25,000 IU/day |
|   Vitamin $B_{12}$ | (12) | 1000 $\mu$g/month IM |
|   Vitamin C | (10) | 100 mg/day |
|   Vitamin E | (12) | ? |
| Intussusception | 2–3 | Surgical repair |
| Hair loss | 3 | Increased dietary protein |
| Gout | 2 | Standard therapy |
| Bowel obstruction due | | |
|   to adhesions | 2 | Surgical repair |
| Pulmonary tuberculosis | 1–4 | Drugs, reversal |
| Peripheral neuromyopathy | Uncommon | TPN |
| Pseudo-obstruction of colon | Uncommon | Antibiotics |

[a] The incidence of complications in the Washington University series is reported in parentheses. When no parentheses are present, the incidence in the Washington University series falls within the range reported in the literature.

The early postoperative complications are those expected in a very obese population: fever, atelectasis, pneumonia, thrombophlebitis, pulmonary embolus, wound infection and wound seroma, and urinary tract infection (2, 4). Cardiopulmonary complications result in an occasional death postoperatively. The problems are similar after gastric bypass, but the importance of some of them varies. Most worrisome initially was the occurrence of anastomotic leaks. The frequency of this complication depends very much on surgical technique, because devascularization of the gastric remnant must not occur. The gastric bypass is a technically more demanding operation. The correct amount of stomach must be left to create a limited reservoir, and a gastric outlet must be created narrow enough to allow slow emptying, but not so narrow as to cause obstruction. In fact, gastric bypass is a controlled outlet obstruction from a small pouch. Chronic vomiting is one of the most common complications after gastric bypass, usually occurring in patients who cannot control their intake postoperatively (Table 1). It is too soon to assess the late complications of gastric bypass. The beneficial results seem at least comparable to those of jejunoileal bypass.

The major complications of jejunoileal bypass that present to the gastroenterologist are the late ones (Table 2). Although it is difficult to estimate, probably over two complications occur per patient, and 30–50% of all patients require postoperative hospitalization at least once (9). The data presented in Tables 2 and 3 are based on the literature and on data from the follow-up of 101 patients from Washington University, St. Louis (courtesy of Drs. J. Halverson, L. Wise, W. F. Ballinger, and G. Zuckerman). Many of the data from the Washington University series are still in the process of analysis. These unpublished data can be referred to only briefly here, but the conclusions or trends will be mentioned where appropriate. Diarrhea is very common, and steatorrhea is nearly universal. Even after 2 years 10–20% of patients still have more than eight stools per day. However, the steatorrhea does not account for all the weight loss, since over half the patients eat fewer calories postoperatively (10). Thus, malnutrition and specific deficiencies arise both from malabsorption and from inadequate intake.

Electrolyte deficiencies are common, and a high percentage of patients require supplementation for potassium, calcium, and magnesium. These ions are lost in the stool. Potassium is reabsorbed in the small intestine and secreted into the colonic lumen. If time for luminal contents in the colon is relatively greater than in the small intestine, as seems likely, potassium loss will be enhanced. Calcium and magnesium deficiency occur because of malabsorption of both dietary and endogenous secretions. The potential losses of calcium are about 1600 mg/day, and for magnesium about 700 mg/day. Moreover, vitamin D malabsorption affects both ions by decreasing absorption. Finally, magnesium replacement is difficult from the diet, because dietary sources (300 mg/day) are not nearly so abundant as the potential losses of this ion. Moreover, the pharmaceutical preparations usually used (MgO) are poorly absorbed and cause diarrhea. Thus, they are avoided by physician and patient. Replacement of potassium should be with potassium citrate, not potassium chloride, since metabolic acidosis usually occurs with severe diarrhea. Calcium carbonate (1–2 g/day or more of calcium) can be used to replace calcium. Calcium carbonate is 40% elemental calcium by weight and is well tolerated by patients. The most satisfactory preparation for magnesium replacement is magnesium gluconate (0.5 g tablets), and frequently as much as 4–6 g/day is required. Most important, hypocalcemia sometimes cannot be corrected until magnesium is replaced.

Severe weakness, usually associated with severe malnutrition, is not uncommon. Sometimes a severe neuromyopathy of the lower extremities, which leads to paresis, is seen (11). This complication can be reversed by total parenteral nutrition, but does not seem to be due to folic acid, vitamin $B_{12}$, or thiamine deficiency.

Renal stones occur frequently after jejunoileal bypass (12). This complication is associated with increased oxalate excretion (4). However, disappointingly, the urinary oxalate excretion cannot be normalized by strict adherence to a low oxalate diet. The addition of oral calcium may prove helpful, but each patient must be monitored for urinary oxalate to determine the proper dose of calcium required, since this will depend on the degree of fat malabsorption (13). Polyarthritis, but more commonly polyarthralgias, can be quite troublesome (14). The usual anti-inflammatory drugs can be useful in therapy, if one remembers to adjust the dose, allowing for drug malabsorption.

Gallstones have also occurred frequently, and have required surgery (9, 15). Other complications requiring surgery include ventral hernias and intussusception (16). Pseudo-obstruction of the bowel occurs in two syndromes according to Bray and colleagues (1, 17). When the small bowel is involved patients present with cramps, diarrhea, and fever. When the colon is involved, distention is the primary symptom. The etiology is thought to be secondary to bacterial overgrowth and is treated with antibiotics effective against anaerobes (e.g., metronidazole 1.5 g/day) (18). All patients after bypass colonize both the small bowel and excluded loop with colonic flora (19). Yet the complication of pseudo-obstruction is quite rare. We have yet to see it at Washington University in our 101 patients. Perhaps other factors, such as overgrowth of a specific toxigenic bacteria, are required for the syndrome, as for the production of antibiotic-associated pseudomembranous colitis.

Liver failure is the most dramatic, but not the most frequent complication. It is the major late complication that leads to death, but other complications can significantly impair the patient's state of health. Liver biopsy changes occur frequently after bypass, especially in the first year postoperatively (20, 21). In our series of patients fat, fibrosis, inflammation, and ballooning degeneration of cells, while present to varying degrees preoperatively, all increase postoperatively. Fibrosis increases from 12% of patients to 33% by 1 year. Hepatic changes that occur uniquely postoperatively include cholestasis and noncaseating granulomata (7%). Most important, fibrosis and cirrhosis have been noted to progress without worsening hepatic function as measured by the usual parameters. Liver biopsy (and perhaps wedged hepatic pressure) must be followed to allow assessment of continuing fibrosis and portal hypertension.

The treatment of hepatic complications is uncertain. It has been suggested that the liver disease is related to protein malnutrition (22) but restoration of normal amino acid patterns in the blood is more striking than clinical improvement after protein feeding. Oral protein feeding is complicated by the existing malabsorption. Hence total parenteral nutrition has been advocated for serious liver disease (23). Although no controlled data are available our experience would suggest that this is a useful form of therapy. Reversal of hepatic dysfunction has been reported with total parenteral feeding and clearly can occur (24). Cirrhosis and death are the final results of progressive liver disease (25). This course usually occurs over the first 12 or 24 months postoperatively. Hence careful monitoring of liver function and liver biopsies should be performed during this period, and perhaps longer.

Vitamin deficiencies may develop and must be searched for. Vitamin $B_{12}$ deficiency can occur despite some residual ileum in the path of food (26). This may be related to the fact that most of the ileal receptors for the intrinsic factor–$B_{12}$ complex are not in the most terminal segment, but in the segments more cephalad, which would be in the bypassed segment (27). Folate deficiency is more common, and anemia, when it occurs, is due to deficiencies of these vitamins plus iron. Replacement of water-soluble vitamins is usually not a problem. Fat-soluble vitamin deficiencies occur frequently and are more of a problem in treatment. Vitamin A and D deficiencies are frequent (28) and deficiency of vitamin D has led to metabolic bone disease (29, 30). Since vitamins A and D require bile acids for solubilization and absorption, treatment with the usual water-insoluble forms of these vitamins is difficult. Vitamin A may be required in doses as high as 25,000–50,000 IU per day. However, serum vitamin A level should be monitored to avoid hypervitaminosis A. Until recently, only fat-soluble vitamin D preparations were available, and were given in an oral dose of 50,000 IU 2–3 times weekly. To detect hypercalcinuria, 24 hour urinary calcium should be checked every 3–6 months. If the excretion is low ($< 50$ mg/day) more vitamin D, calcium, or both are needed. On a 1500 mg calcium intake (assuming 33% malabsorption) urinary excretions should be in the range of 100–200 mg. Repletion with vitamin D can be monitored by following 25-OH vitamin D levels. Although 1,25-$(OH)_2$ vitamin D is now available, it is approved only for use in uremia. It is not known what dose of this water-soluble vitamin will be needed in bypass patients, but 0.25 $\mu$g/day is the lowest available dose. When this begins to be used, careful monitoring of serum and urinary calcium will be needed to avoid toxicity.

Pulmonary tuberculosis occurs occasionally after bypass (31). Treatment again is difficult and uncertain because of the malabsorption of antituberculosis drugs. Although most studies do not mention the onset of psychiatric disease after bypass, we have noticed this complication in 7% of our patients. Depression was the most common diagnosis, but anxiety neurosis and alcoholism also developed.

It is obvious that the diagnosis and management of these multiple complications require an understanding, cooperative, mentally sound patient, and an interested, patient, and knowledgeable physician. Moreover, not all complications have been listed; for example, dermatoses and zinc deficiency could be discussed. Finally, although the most dramatic complications occur within the first 24 months, problems continue for 5–7 years. Among 70 patients in our series who still have their bypass intact (mean postoperative time of 50 months), over three-quarters have shown some increase in weight from their nadir, and about half have regained a mean of 9% of their *original* weight. Electrolyte depletion and hypovitaminosis persist in 10–20% of patients. Hence continuous care of these patients is needed.

Despite the best of care, many patients will require reanastomosis because of complications (Table 3). We have had to reverse 25% of our patients (32). The most common reasons for reversal in our series were severe electrolyte deficiencies, or malnutrition and profound weakness, often in combination. Liver disease was another major reason for reversal. No patient was reversed only for neurological or psychiatric symptoms, but these were frequent. Parenteral nutrition has been helpful in reversing some of the hepatic dysfunction also, but has not been used as definitive therapy. Total parenteral nutrition has been used to improve hepatic function prior to reanastomosis. At present, indications for reanastomosis for jejunoileal bypass should include: (*a*) hepatic failure (encephalopathy, onset of cirrhosis, increasing hyperbilirubinemia), (*b*) worsening hepatic fibrosis, (*c*) weight loss to below ideal weight (revision rather than reanastomosis should be considered here if malnutrition

Table 3    Reasons for Reanastomosis[a]

| Complications | Number of Patients | Primary Reason for Reversal |
|---|---|---|
| Worsening liver function | 10 | 5 |
| Malnutrition/weakness | 15 | 6 |
| Electrolyte deficiency | 7 | 5 |
| Arthralgias | 6 | 2 |
| Protracted vomiting | 2 | 2 |
| Abdominal pain | 6 | 1 |
| Alcoholism | 1 | 1 |
| Tuberculosis | 2 | 1 |
| Renal failure | 1 | 1 |
| Pneumoperitoneum | 1 | 1 |
| Neurological symptoms | 7 | 0 |
| Psychiatric illness | 5 | 0 |

[a] Washington University series, 25 patients.

is not marked), (d) debilitating weakness, (e) severe psychiatric problems, (f) intractable electrolyte deficiency, and (g) pulmonary tuberculosis.

In the Washington University series of 101 patients there have been 5% late deaths and a reversal rate of 25% (23 patients remain alive, 2 died). Of the patients that remain alive with bypass intact, about half are having significant problems, such as recurrent urinary tract stones and recurrent hospitalizations for electrolyte deficiencies and other problems.

Even when the operations are restricted in number, the frequency and severity of complications after jejunoileal bypass is such that this operation should rarely, if ever, be performed. It is too early to reach conclusions about gastric bypass, but this procedure seems initially to have a higher benefit : risk ratio. With recent technical modification (e.g., use of staples, not dividing the stomach), gastric bypass can be more safely performed. It is still a procedure that requires much surgical experience.

If gastric bypass is to be considered, we must carefully rethink our criteria for acceptance for this operation. It is not known if this procedure will prolong life or decrease the incidence of vascular complications. In particular, it is not enough to show absence of preexisting diagnosable psychiatric disease, but the patients should be emotionally stable enough to maintain close physician contact, should have shown they were able to maintain a stable life-style and follow a diet and instructions in the past, and should not be severely compulsive overeaters. Their emotional problems will not disappear with the bypass and their overeating will lead to chronic nausea and vomiting in a few cases which may not be amenable to treatment postoperatively.

Since the gastric bypass cannot be reversed so easily as the jejunoileal bypass, the procedure should be done with great caution. Since the proper role of surgery in the management of obesity is not yet clear, it is the responsibility of the medical profession to proceed with gastric bypass surgery in a small number of centers that can carefully follow and report on all their patients, so that an accurate long-term assessment of the procedure can be obtained. Moreover, adaptation (i.e., enlargement of the stoma) could possibly occur with time. Such adaptation is the cause of the multiplicity of gastric procedures for obesity to date. Our experience with late weight gain in jejunoileal bypass, though for different reasons, makes us cautious about premature optimism for gastric bypass surgery.

Whichever operation is performed for obesity, it is essential to monitor the vitamin and mineral status of the patients carefully for an extended period of time, and perhaps indefinitely. Certain vitamin deficiencies (A and D) may not become apparent for a number of years and continued surveillance will be required.

# REFERENCES

1. G. A. Bray, *The Obese Patient*, Saunders, Philadelphia, 1976.
2. L. Wise, "Iatrogenic Short Bowel Syndrome: Surgical Treatment of Morbid Exogenous Obesity, Chapter 7 in W. F. Ballinger and T. Drapanas, Eds., *Practice of Surgery*, Vol. II, Mosby, St. Louis, 1975.
3. S. J. Young, D. H. Alpers, C. C. Norland, and R. A. Woodruff, Psychiatric illness and the irritable bowel syndrome, *Gastroenterology*, **70**, 162 (1976).
4. J. D. Halverson, L. Wise, M. F. Wazna, and W. F. Ballinger, Jejunoileal bypass for morbid obesity. A critical appraisal, *Am. J. Med.*, **64**, 461 (1978).
5. P. Davis and J. Hahn-Pedersen, Improvement in quality of life following jejunoileal bypass surgery for obesity, *Scand. J. Gastroenterology*, **12**, 769 (1977).
6. C. Solow, Psychological aspects of intestinal bypass surgery for massive obesity: Current status, *Am. J. Clin. Nutr.*, **30**, 103, (1977).
7. E. E. Mason, K. J. Printen, C. E. Hartford, and W. C. Boyd, Optimizing results of gastric bypass, *Ann. Surg.*, **182**, 405 (1975).
8. A. S. Hermrich, W. R. Jewell, and C. A. Hardin, Gastric bypass for morbid obesity. Results and complications, *Surgery*, **80**, 498 (1976).
9. G. A. Bray, R. E. Barry, J. R. Benfield, et al., Intestinal bypass operation as a treatment for obesity, *Ann. Int. Med.*, **85**, 97 (1976).
10. S. C. Condon, N. J. Jones, L. Wise, and D. H. Alpers, Role of caloric intake in the weight loss after jejunoileal bypass for obesity, *Gastroenterology*, **74**, 34 (1978).
11. A. K. Ciongoli and C. M. Poser, Fat malabsorption neuromyopathy, *Arch. Neurol.*, **26**, 402 (1972).

12. J. P. O'Leary, W. K. Thomas, and E. R. Woodward, Urinary tract stone after small bowel bypass for morbid obesity, *Am. J. Surg.* **127,** 142 (1974).

13. D. E. Barilla, C. Notz, D. Kennedy, and C. Y. C. Pak, Renal oxalate excretion following oral oxalate loads in patients with ileal disease and with renal and absorptive hypercalcemia, *Am. J. Med.,* **64,** 579 (1978).

14. J. R. Wands, J. T. Lamont, E. Mann, and K. J. Isselbacher, Arthritis associated with intestinal bypass procedures for morbid obesity, *New Engl. J. Med.,* **294,** 123 (1976).

15. J. M. Campbell, T. K. Hunt, J. H. Karam, P. H. Forsham, Jejunoileal bypass as a treatment for morbid obesity, *Arch. Int. Med.,* **137,** 602 (1977).

16. L. T. DeWind and J. H. Payne, Intestinal bypass surgery for morbid obesity, *J.A.M.A.,* **236,** 2298 (1976).

17. R. E. Barry, J. R. Manfield, and G. A. Bray, Colonic pseudoobstruction: A new complication of jejunoileal bypass, *Gut,* **16,** 903 (1975).

18. W. W. Faloon, Ileal bypass for obesity: post-operative perspective, *Hospital Practice,* January 1977, p. 73.

19. P. Conodi, P. A. Wideman, V. L. Sutter, et al., Bacterial flora of the small bowel before and after bypass procedure for morbid obesity, *J. Inf. Dis.,* **137,** 1 (1978).

20. R. L. Peters, T. Gay, and T. B. Reynolds, Post jejunoileal bypass hepatic disease: its similarity to alcohol hepatic disease, *Am. J. Clin. Path.* **63,** 318 (1975).

21. W. H. Kern, J. H. Payne, and L. T. DeWind, Hepatic changes after small intestinal bypass for morbid obesity, *Am. J. Clin. Pathol.,* **61,** 763 (1974).

22. R. T. Moxley, T. Pozefsky, and D. H. Lockwood, Protein nutrition and liver disease after jejunoileal bypass for morbid obesity, *New Engl. J. Med.,* **290,** 721 (1974).

23. A. L. Baker, Nutrition and liver disease: managing the hepatic complications of jejunoileal bypass surgery, *Practical Gastroenterology,* January/February 1978, p. 19.

24. F. C. Ames, D. E. M. Copeland, D. C. Leak, et al., Liver dysfunction following small bowel bypass for obesity: non-operative treatment of fatty metamorphosis with parenteral hyperalimentation, *J.A.M.A.,* **235,** 1249 (1976).

25. J. C. Mangla, W. Hoy, Y. Kin, and M. Chopek, Cirrhosis and death after jejunoileal shunt for obesity, *Am. J. Dig. Dis.,* **19,** 759 (1974).

26. E. Juhl, A. Brunsgaard, B. Hippe, et al., Vitamin $B_{12}$ depletion in obese patients treated with jejunoileal shunt, *Scand. J. Gastroenterology,* **9,** 534 (1974).

27. C. H. Hagedorn and D. H. Alpers, Distribution of intrinsic factor-vitamin $B_{12}$ receptors in human intestine, *Gastroenterology,* **73,** 1019 (1977).

28. S. L. Teitelbaum, J. D. Halverson, M. Bates, et al., Abnormalities of circulating 25-OH vitamin D after jejunal-ileal bypass for obesity, *Ann. Int. Med.,* **86,** 289 (1977).

29. A. M. Parfitt, M. J. Miller, B. Frame, et al., Metabolic bone disease after intestinal bypass for treatment of obesity, *Ann. Int. Med.,* **89,** 193 (1978).

30. J. D. Halverson, S. L. Teitelbaum, J. G. Haddad, and W. A. Murphy, Skeletal abnormalities after jejunoileal bypass, *Ann. Surg.,* in press, 1978.

31. R. M. Bruce and L. Wise, Tuberculosis after jejunoileal bypass for obesity, *Ann. Int. Med.,* **87,** 574 (1977).

32. J. D. Halverson, K. Gentry, L. Wise, and W. F. Ballinger, Reanastomosis after jejunoileal bypass, *Surgery,* **84,** 241 (1978).

# Effect of Altered Nutrition on the Gastrointestinal Tract

# 13

# Early Nutrition and Intestinal Adaptation

STEVEN M. SCHWARZ, M.D., AND
WILLIAM C. HEIRD, M.D.

Columbia University College of Physicians and Surgeons, New York, New York

The most general definition of the term adaptation is a change in structure, function, or form that produces better adjustment to the environment. In gastroenterology, however, adaptation is defined more specifically. The changes that take place in the remaining intestine following intestinal resection are called adaptive changes. Following colonic resection, for example, the ileum assumes some of the colonic functions (1); similarly, following jejunal resection the ileum assumes jejunal function (2), and following ileal resection the jejunum assumes some of the functions of the ileum (3). Another specific gastroenterological definition of adaptation refers to the changes in function that occur in response to diet, particularly the alterations that result as a response to specific dietary components.

Before discussing adaptive changes in response to diet during development, it is useful to review the general information concerning this aspect of intestinal adaptation—specifically, the general role of feeding in maintenance of intestinal mucosal mass and the effects of specific nutrients on mucosal enzyme activities.

## ROLE OF FEEDING IN MAINTENANCE OF INTESTINAL MUCOSAL MASS

The intestinal mucosal mass decreases with starvation (4, 5), but whether this decrease is a function merely of the cessation of enteral intake or reflects an altered nutritional status is not clear. For example, the muco-

sal mass of animals in which nutritional status is maintained with parenteral nutrients decreases by approximately 50% (6, 7), the same magnitude
observed in animals that receive only water (7). However, the decrease in
mucosal mass occurs during the first 3 days of parenteral nutrition, with
no change in mass thereafter (8); in contrast, mucosal mass decreases
continuously in starved animals (7). Such studies suggest that the absence of enteral feedings, with or without a change in nutritional status,
results in a decreased mucosal mass but that the magnitude of this decrease is greater under conditions of starvation, perhaps because of alterations in nutritional status.

A number of possible mechanisms have been proposed to explain the
observed atrophic effect of starvation or lack of enterally supplied nutrients on enteric tissues. Since intestinal epithelium has a high mitotic
index (8) and consequently high nitrogen and energy requirements, the
disproportionate effect of undernutrition on mucosal integrity (9) is
easily understood. However, as noted above, enteral intake per se may
be necessary for maintenance of the small intestinal mass (10, 11). One
explanation for the requirement for enteral intake is based on the fact
that certain gastrointestinal hormones which exert trophic effects on intestinal epithelium are diminished in the absence of oral feedings. It is
well known that gastrin, secreted by antral mucosa, exerts positive trophic
effects on intestinal tissues. Johnson and co-workers have shown that both
serum and antral gastrin levels are significantly lower in starved animals
(12) as well as in animals maintained solely with parenteral nutrients
(13), and that pharmacologic doses of pentagastrin prevent the observed
decrease in intestinal mucosal mass of parenterally fed animals (14).

Other gastrointestinal hormones that may exert trophic effects on the
bowel, such as cholecystokinin (15) and enteroglucagon (16), are also
suppressed during fasting.

The fact that these gastrointestinal hormones seem to exert positive
trophic effects on intestinal epithelium raises the question of whether the
observed actions are primary or are manifested through intermediary
agents. One possible explanation is that pancreatic or biliary secretions,
or both, which are released by gut hormones, may be the active factors for
maintenance of intestinal epithelial mass. Altman and Leblond demonstrated that villus height of isolated duodenal segments of the rat decreased when the duodenal papilla was excluded (17) and that trans-
plantation of the papilla to isolated ileal segments in the dog resulted
in marked ileal villus enlargement (18). Further, bile diversion had no
effect on the observed ileal hypertrophy, suggesting that pancreatic secretions contained the apparent trophic factor. More recently, however,
Roy and co-workers (19) observed that bile diversion from the rat intesti-

Table 1    Effect of Dietary Carbohydrate on Intestinal Disacchridase Activities[a]

| Carbohydrate | Effect |
| --- | --- |
| Sucrose | Increased sucrase, maltase |
| Fructose | Increased sucrase, maltase |
| Glucose | Increased, sucrase, maltase($\pm$) |
| Lactose | None |
| Galactose | None |
| Maltose | None |

[a] Data adapted by authors from Rosensweig (20) and Rosensweig and Herman (21, 22).

nal lumen resulted within 48 hours in villous hypoplasia of the ileum. Subsequent perfusion of the intestine with sodium taurocholate reversed these changes, suggesting that bile salts exert important regulatory influences on enterocyte kinetics.

These seemingly discrepant studies raise a number of questions about the relative roles of pancreatic and biliary secretions in the growth of intestinal epithelium. If all the aforementioned results are to be accepted, it seems that species differences, differential effects on duodenal versus ileal mucosa, or both, must be postulated.

## EFFECT OF SPECIFIC NUTRIENTS ON MUCOSAL ENZYME ACTIVITIES

In contrast to the general effect of enteral intake on mucosal mass is the effect of specific nutrients on mucosal enzyme activities. The effects of dietary carbohydrates demonstrated in both adult human volunteers and adult animals are summarized in Table 1 (20–22). Sucrose feeding results in an increased specific activity of intestinal sucrase and a smaller increase in intestinal maltase (21). Both dietary fructose (20, 21) and glucose (22) also result in increased sucrase and maltase activities. Although increase in intestinal lactase activity in response to lactose feeding has been reported (23), most studies suggest that intestinal lactase activity does not respond to ingestion of either lactose or other carbohydrates (24–26). Dietary carbohydrates also increase the activities of several intracellular glycolytic enzymes (27, 28). For example, dietary glucose results in increased activity of the intracellular enzymes con-

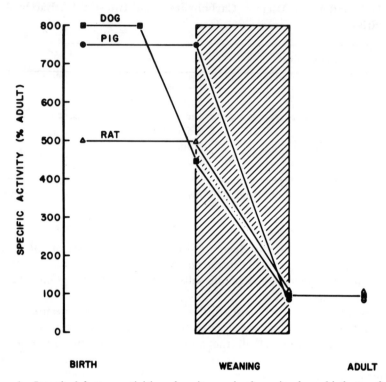

**Figure 1.** Intestinal lactase activities of various animal species from birth to adulthood. [Adapted by the authors from data of Goldstein and co-workers Aumaitre and Corring (32), and Welsh and Walter (33).]

cerned with glucose metabolism whereas dietary fructose and galactose result in increased activities of the intracellular enzymes involved in fructose and galactose metabolism, respectively. These changes also occur in response to enteral but not parenteral folic acid (29) and steroid hormones (30).

## DEVELOPMENTAL CHANGES IN INTESTINAL ENZYME ACTIVITIES

The period immediately following birth is characterized by dramatic physiological activity as the newborn animal adapts to an extrauterine existence. For many years, it has been known that this environmental change is accompanied by marked developmental alterations of the pul-

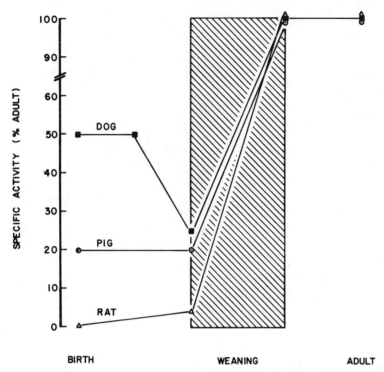

**Figure 2.** Intestinal sucrase activities of various animal species from birth to adult-hood. [Adapted by the authors from data of Goldstein and co-workers (31), Aumaitre Corring (32), and Welsh and Walker (33).]

monary and cardiovascular systems. More recently, developmental changes of a similar magnitude have been found to occur in the new-born gastrointestinal tract. For ethical as well as technical reasons, these developmental studies have been conducted largely in laboratory animals. Information about the development of the human intestine, particularly information about the role of intraluminal nutrients in the morphologic and enzymatic adaptation of the intestine to extrauterine life, is sparse.

The normal developmental pattern of lactase and sucrase activities in several animal species is outlined in Figures 1 and 2 (31–33). At birth, most species have lactase activities far in excess of normal adult values and little, if any, sucrase activity. These hydrolase activities correspond to the diet of the preweaning animal, in which lactose is the only carbohydrate. At the time of weaning lactose activity drops precipitously while sucrase (and maltase) activity increases dramatically, presumably

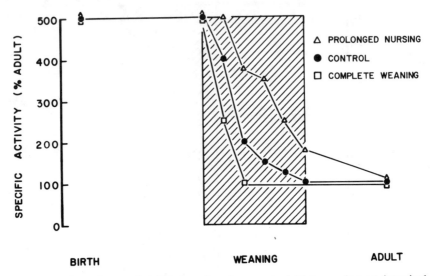

**Figure 3.** Effect of normal (–O–), late (–△–), or early (–□–) weaning on intestinal lactase activity in the rat. [Adapted by the authors from data of Goldstein and co-workers (31), and Lebenthal and co-workers (34).]

also an adaptive change which allows the animal to tolerate a diet containing a variety of carbohydrates other than lactose.

Attempts to modify this developmental pattern by dietary manipulation suggest that these changes occur prior to and regardless of a change in diet. Lebenthal and co-workers (34) determined lactase and sucrase activities of suckling rats that were either allowed to complete the normal weaning cycle or suckled for an extended period (Figures 3 and 4). The developmental decline in lactase specific activity occurred despite the extended period of suckling; however, the decline was less precipitous. Despite the absence of dietary sucrose, the developmental increment in sucrase activity was virtually unaffected by prolonged suckling (Figure 4). Goldstein and co-workers (31) demonstrated a precocious increase in sucrase activity as well as a precocious decline in lactase activity with early complete weaning, but the basic developmental pattern remained intact.

Such studies suggest that the intestinal epithelium of newborn animals is "preprogrammed" to undergo a specific pattern of development with respect to sugar hydrolase activities and that dietary influences are of little if any importance. Recent studies of Koldovsky and co-workers (35) support this concept. These investigators found that sucrase activity of fetal rat jejunum transplanted beneath the renal capsule of adult rats

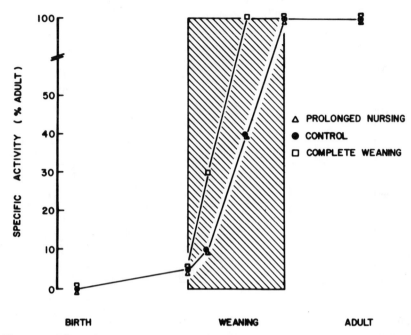

**Figure 4.** Effect of normal (–O–), late (–△–), or early (–□–) weaning on intestinal sucrase activity of the rat. [Adapted by the authors from data of Goldstein and co-workers (31), and Lebenthal and co-workers (34).]

increased normally. The only explanations for such an increase without the direct effect of intraluminal nutrients are that the newborn small intestinal epitheleum is preprogrammed to undergo specific developmental changes or that factors other than diet mediate these changes (e.g., hormones or other blood-borne factors).

## EFFECT OF TYPE OF FEEDING ON INTESTINAL DEVELOPMENT

There is yet another aspect of the effect of nutrients on small intestinal development that must be discussed. This stems from an observation by Widdowson and co-workers (36) about growth of the small intestine of piglets during the first 24 hours of life (Figure 5). The intestine of the suckled piglets, in contrast to the intestine of those that received only water, showed a marked increase in weight during this interval. This increased weight was due primarily to growth of the jejunum and the ileum. Jejunal growth was limited almost entirely to the mucosal por-

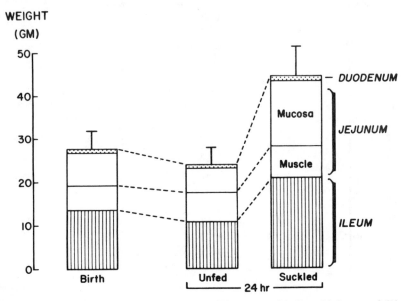

**Figure 5.** Growth of the small intestine of piglets over the first 24 hours of life. [Adapted by the authors from data of Widdowson and co-workers (36).]

tion, with the jejunal mucosal mass of these animals 90% greater than that of animals at birth.

The question of whether this growth was due solely to feeding or specifically to feeding natural milk obviously arises. Our comparison of the growth of the small intestine of beagle puppies over the first 24 hours of life as a function of type of feeding (i.e., left with their mothers and allowed to suckle ad lib or separated from the mothers and fed artificially) provides some insight into this question (37). Although body, kidney, and liver weights of the two groups were similar, the weight of the small intestine of the suckled group was 75% greater than that of the group fed artificially. This increased intestinal mass was due entirely to differences in mucosal mass; the weight of the nonmucosal portion of the small intestine was similar in the two groups. Despite the marked difference in mucosal weight there was no difference in disaccharidase activities between the two groups.

This study strongly suggests that the colostrum of the dog contains a factor that exerts a specific growth stimulatory effect on the small intestinal mucosa. This evidence for such a factor in the dog and the possibility of such a factor in the pig (36) suggests that colostrum, and perhaps milk, of all animal species might contain a factor that stimulates growth of intestinal mucosa. In fact, Klagsbrun and co-workers (38) have shown that the milk of a number of animal species contains a small protein which stimulates growth of fibroblasts in vitro. The relationship between this factor and the increased intestinal mucosal growth of suckled beagle puppies remains to be established.

## REFERENCES

1. A. W. Wilkinson, *Mod. Prob. Petiatr.*, **11**, 191 (1968).
2. D. W. Wilmore, *J. Pediatr.*, **80**, 88 (1972).
3. W. F. Young, et al., *Arch. Dis. Child.*, **44**, 465 (1969).
4. L. K. McNeill and J. R. Hamilton, *Pediatr.*, **47**, 65 (1971).
5. J. P. A. McManus and K. J. Isselbacher, *Gastroenterology*, **59**, 214 (1970).
6. W. C. Heird et al., *Gastroenterology*, **66**, A55 (1974).
7. W. C. Heird, unpublished observations.
8. F. D. Bertalanffy and K. P. Nagy, *Acta Anat.*, **45**, 362 (1961).
9. M. Steiner et al., *Am. J. Physiol.*, **215**, 75 (1968).
10. E. J. Feldman et al., *Gastroenterology*, **70**, 712 (1976).
11. L. D. Dworkin et al., *Gastroenterology*, **71**, 626 (1976).
12. L. Lichtenberger, J. D. Welsh, and L. R. Johnson, *Am. J. Dig. Dis.*, **21**, 33 (1976).
13. L. R. Johnson et al., *Gastroenterology*, **68**, 1177 (1975).
14. L. R. Johnson et al., *Gastroenterology*, **68**, 1184 (1975).
15. L. R. Johnson and P. Guthrie, *Gastroenterology*, **70**, 1965 (1976).
16. M. D. Rudo and H. Rosenberg, *Proc. Soc. Exp. Biol. Med.*, **142**, 521 (1973).
17. G. G. Altman and C. P. Leblond, *Am. J. Anat.*, **127**, 15 (1970).
18. G. G. Altman and C. P. Leblond, *Am. J. Anat.*, **132**, 167 (1971).
19. C. C. Roy et al., *Proc. Soc. Exp. Biol. Med.*, **149**, 1000 (1975).
20. N. S. Rosensweig, *Am. J. Clin. Nutr.*, **28**, 648 (1975).
21. N. S. Rosensweig and R. H. Herman, *J. Clin. Invest.*, **47**, 2253 (1968).
22. N. S. Rosensweig and R. H. Herman, *Am. J. Clin. Nutr.*, **23**, 1373 (1970).
23. G. D. Cain et al., *Scand. J. Gastroenterology*, **4**, 545 (1969).
24. G. T. Keusch et al., *Am. J. Clin. Nutr.*, **22**, 638 (1969).
25. P. Cuatrecasas et al., *Lancet*, **1**, 14 (1965).
26. T. Gilat et al., *Gastroenterology*, **62**, 1125 (1972).
27. F. B. Stifel et al., *Biochim. Biophys. Acta*, **170**, 221 (1968).
28. N. S. Rosensweig et al., *Biochim. Biophys. Acta*, **170**, 223 (1963).
29. N. S. Rosensweig, R. H. Herman, and F. B. Stifel, *Biochim. Biophys. Acta*, **208**, 373 (1970).
30. F. B. Stifel et al., *Biochim. Biophys. Acta*, **208**, 368 (1970).
31. R. Goldstein et al., *Am. J. Clin. Nutr.*, **24**, 1224 (1971).
32. A. Aumaitre and T. Corring, *Nutr. Metab.*, **22**, 244 (1978).

33. J. B. Welsh and A. Walker, *Proc. Soc. Exp. Biol. Med.,* **120,** 525 (1965).

34. E. Lebenthal, J. Sunshine, and N. Kretchmer, *Gastroenterology,* **64,** 1136 (1973).

35. O. Koldovsky et al., *Pediatr. Res.,* **12,** 438 (1978).

36. E. M. Widdowson, V. E. Colombo, and C. A. Artavanis, *Biol. Neonate,* **28,** 272 (1976).

37. W. C. Heird and I. H. Hansen *Pediatr. Res.,* **11,** 406 (1977).

38. M. Klagsbrun, *Proc. Natl. Acad. Sci.,* **75,** 5057 (1978).

# 14

# Cellular and Immune Changes in the Gastrointestinal Tract in Malnutrition

W. ALLAN WALKER, M.D.

Harvard Medical School and Massachusetts General Hospital, Boston, Massachusetts

An important adaptation of the gastrointestinal tract to the external environment is the development of a mucosal barrier against the penetration of harmful substances (bacteria and viruses, toxins, and antigens) present within the intestinal lumen. The fully developed and functional gastrointestinal tract must be prepared to deal with continuous colonization of the gut by bacteria, the formation of toxic byproducts of bacteria and viruses (enterotoxins and endotoxins), and the ingestion of antigens (milk proteins). These potentially noxious substances, if allowed to penetrate the mucosal epithelial barrier in pathologic quantities, can cause inflammatory and allergic reactions that may result in gastrointestinal and systemic disease states (1).

To combat the potential danger of invasion across the mucosal barrier, man has developed an elaborate system of defense mechanisms within the lumen and on the luminal mucosal surface which act to control and maintain the epithelium as an impermeable barrier to the uptake of macromolecular antigens. These defenses include the unique local immunologic system adapted to function in the complicated milieu of the intestine, as well as other nonimmunologic processes, such as a gastric barrier, intestinal surface proteins, peristaltic movement, and natural antibacterial substances (lysozyme and the bile salts), which work in cooperation to provide maximum protection for the intestinal surface (2). Unfortunately, at times when primary malnutrition exists, particularly with protein-calorie malnutrition, this elaborate local defense system is disrupted. As a result of disruption of the mucosal barrier, malnourished individuals are particularly vulnerable to pathologic penetration of harmful intraluminal substances. The consequences of altered host defense are susceptibility to infection, potential for hypersensitivity reactions, and formation of circulating immune complexes. With these reactions comes the potential for developing life-threatening secondary diseases, such as bacterial gastroenteritis, sepsis, arthritis, nephritis, and hepatitis. Fortunately, nature has provided a means for potential passive protection of the vulnerable malnourished individual, which can provide a short-term passive protective role against the dangers of a deficient intestinal defense system. This substance, human milk, might potentially be used in the treatment of these individuals.

In this review of alterations and cellular and immune functions of the gastrointestinal tract in malnutrition, the normal adaptations of host protection in the hostile intraluminal environment will be reviewed. A brief synopsis of the uniqueness of the local immune system on mucosal surfaces providing an immune exclusion of intestinal antigens will also be set forth. The derangement in gastrointestinal structure and function in malnutrition will be reviewed, as well as the consistent immunologic deficits reported in both malnourished human patients and malnourished animal models, and finally, the consequences of malnutrition and its effect on the mucosal barrier will be considered. Theoretical rehabilitation measures that provide a means of combating this nutritional deficit and preventing the secondary life-threatening complication of altered host defense will be presented.

## GUT ADAPTATIONS FOR HOST DEFENSE

### Concept in Mucosal Barrier

In order to function optimally as a digestive organ, the small intestine has evolved by various adaptations to an enormous surface area roughly equivalent to that of a singles tennis court. This surface area must provide the basis for end stages of digestion and also is the site for transport of nutrients into the systemic circulation. The surface is also in direct contact with an external environment and as such must be in constant vigilance against penetration of foreign substances that can cause adverse reactions within the host. In order for the gastrointestinal tract to function adequately as a mucosal barrier, the functional unit of the small intestine, the crypt–villus unit, must operate optimally. Under normal physiologic conditions cells are continuously proliferating within the crypt region and migrating up the villus surface towards the villus tip. In the process of migration, these cells evolve from an undifferentiated state to highly differentiated epithelial cells which are especially adapted not only for absorption but also for mucosal barrier function. Of particular importance is the microvillus and glycocalyx on the luminal surface of the columnar epithelial cell. This compartment provides an active metabolic site for host barrier function. The functional microvillus surface is completely replaced in man every 3 days. For this turnover process to operate optimally, a continued source of exogenous energy, particularly protein calories, must be provided to the host. Furthermore, the energy source seems to be best suited for intestinal maintenance if it is provided by an enteric route (3, 4). It would appear that some nutrients absorbed across the intestinal epithelial surface are necessary for supplying energy to replenish the mucosal epithelium.

### Techniques for Measuring Cellular Turnover in Migration and Maturation of Intestinal Cell Surface

Numerous experimental techniques have been devised to quantitate cell turnover, cell migration, and cell maturation to determine if the gut is functioning physiologically. These techniques used in vitro as intestinal organ cell cultures of human biopsy material or used in vivo as experimental animal models have been most helpful in defining the functional and physiologic aberrations associated with various malnutritional states. The most commonly used technique is the uptake and incorporation of $^3$H-thymidine into intestinal cells (5). Tritiated thymidine is injected into animals or infused into the incubation media of organ or cell cultures and the amount of radioactivity within the epithelium is determined. The amount of radioactivity in epithelial cells is proportional to the number of new cells formed and is used to determine cell turnover. Under conditions where cells are proliferating in a normal or at an increased rate there is either a normal or an increased amount of radioactivity in the mucosal homogenates of these cells. Under conditions where cell turnover has decreased, there is decreased radioactivity. Using a radioautographic modification of the $^3$H-thymidine incorporation, one can determine not only the amount of radioactivity but the progression of radioactivity in cells as these cells migrate from the crypt into the intestinal villus (6). Under conditions of decreased migration, there is a decrease in the number of radioactive particles present in cells within the crypt–villus unit per unit time. Under conditions of increased migration, these cells containing radioactive material reach the villus tip in a shorter time. In order to assess the maturation of epithelial cells, scrapings and homogenates of these cells are obtained and assayed for specific marker enzymes. Brush border marker enzymes, including the disaccharidases such as sucrase and alkaline phosphatase, have been used as a quantitative assessment of mature cells (7). Enzymes such as thymidine kinase have been used as a marker for crypt cells and as such have been used to quantitate the number of immature crypt cells in any intestinal preparation. A ratio of these two enzymatic activities is an important measure of the degree of mature versus immature intestinal surface that exists. These types of studies will be mentioned as we consider aberrations in intestinal function in malnutrition.

## MACROMOLECULAR TRANSPORT—PHYSIOLOGIC UPTAKE AND LOCAL IMMUNE RESPONSE

### Macromolecular Transport in the Gut

In combined morphologic studies, the small intestinal epithelial cell can be demonstrated to engulf macromolecular intraluminal antigens by an endocytotic process indistinguishable from the pinocytosis process described in human macrophages (Figure 1) (8). The initial event in this process is an interaction between large molecules within the intestinal lumen and components of the microvillus membrane of intestinal absorptive cell (adsorption). In order for these molecules to interact with the microvillus, they must escape intraluminal proteolysis and migrate to the active glycocalyx compartment, which contains antibodies and other enzymes that can potentially break them down. When a sufficient concentration of molecules comes in contact with the cell membrane, invagination occurs and small vesicles are formed. After invagination, antigens migrate within membrane-bound vesicles (phagosomes) to the supranuclear region of the cell where vesicles coalesce with lysosomes to form large vacuoles (phagolysosomes). Within these structures, intracellular digestion occurs. However, small quantities of ingested molecules escape breakdown and migrate to the basal surface of the cell to be deposited in the interstitial space by a reversal of the pinocytosis process. Under normal physiologic conditions, macrophages present in the lamina propria of the small intestine interact with these antigens as a second line of defense against the penetration of antigen into the circulation. When excessive quantities of antigens traverse the intestinal epithelial cell, or when secondary defenses are lacking or diminished, as in secondary IgA deficiency, antigens may diffuse into the interstitial space and enter the systemic circulation. The penetration of foreign antigens into the circulation may in turn evoke allergic and toxigenic reactions manifested by disease states (1).

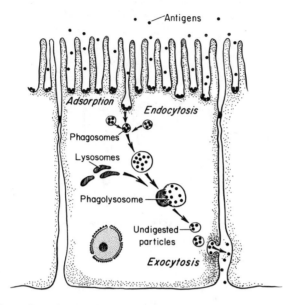

**Figure 1.** General mechanism for the uptake and transport of antigens by the intestinal epithelial cell. After macromolecular antigens adhere to the microvillus membrane (adsorption), invagination of the membrane (endocytosis) occurs and small vesicles are formed. Vesicles migrate toward the center of the cell and combine to form larger vacuoles (phagosomes). Intracellular digestion occurs when lysosomes (containing proteolytic enzymes) combine with phagosomes to form phagolysosomes. Intact antigens that remain after digestion are deposited in the interstitial space by a reverse endocytosis (exocytosis). [From Walker and Isselbacher (1).]

Several clinical studies suggest that macromolecules can cross the mucosal barrier under normal physiologic conditions in man (1, 2). Since the pinocytosis process of antigen absorption most likely represents a residual of some primitive absorptive mechanism within the alimentary canal (8), the capacity to absorb large molecules may very well be enhanced under conditions where excessive immature small intestine exists. In the absence of the mature microvillus surface and the glycocalyx, antigens may interact with the intestinal surface to a greater extent and potentially could be absorbed in larger quantities and thereby gain access to the systemic circulation. In fact, this observation is supported by evidence suggesting that premature newborn infants can absorb greater quantities of ingested food antigens than older infants or adults (8). Rothberg (9), for example, has measured bovine serum albumin (BSA) in the serum of premature infants fed quantities of that protein normally present in the daily milk requirement. In contrast, circulating BSA

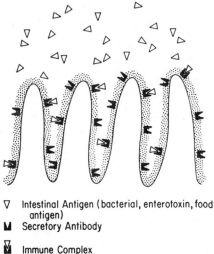

▽    Intestinal Antigen (bacterial, enterotoxin, food
      antigen)
◢    Secretory Antibody

◢    Immune Complex

**Figure 2.** Immune exclusion at the surface of the gastrointestinal tract. Intestinal antibodies within the glycocalyx compartment of the intestinal surface interact with antigens, enterotoxins, and bacteria to prevent their attachment to epithelial cell membranes and thereby inhibit antigen uptake by enterocytes. Formation of antigen–antibody complexes on the surface of the small intestine facilitates the operation of other nonimmunologic host defense mechanisms in clearly pathologic substances from the intestine. [From Walker and Isselbacher (12).]

could not be detected in serum samples from older infants fed equivalent quantities of protein. He and others (10, 11) have also reported an increased percentage of infants with the serum samples containing antibodies to food antigens, suggesting that food proteins are absorbed intact into the circulation of these infants in sufficient quantities to evoke a systemic immune response. This same observation has been made in patients with primary malnutrition. It is therefore presumed because of evidence of an immature gastrointestinal tract and the indirect evidence of antigen transport that this same population of patients might have an enhancement of antigen transport under pathologic conditions. Obviously more extensive studies must be done to substantiate this observation. These consequences of alteration in intestinal surface will be discussed in detail later.

## Local Immune Response

An important, if not the most important, component of host defense at the epithelial surface is the presence of intestinal antibodies (12). These antibodies control bacterial proliferation, neutralize viruses, and prevent penetration of endotoxins and intestinal antigens. A deficiency in local intestinal antibodies can severely impair mucosal barrier function, resulting in uptake of noxious substances that can contribute to the pathogenesis of intestinal systemic disease. Although a number of mechanisms of action have been suggested, including opsinization and complement fixation, there is now substantial evidence that a major function of intestinal antibodies is the process of immune exclusion at the mucosal surface. Figure 2 shows a conceptual interpretation of this phenomenon.

Several specific properties of primary secretory antibodies enhance their effectiveness within the gastrointestinal tract. After transport from the lamina propria onto the intestinal surface, secretory antibodies are retained in the mucus coat on the surface of the epithelial cells by interaction with cystine residues contained in mucins present within the glycocalyx. This stationary location of antibodies in juxtaposition to the intestinal epithelial cell allows for more effective interaction with intestinal antigens coming in contact with the mucosal surface. This property of secretory antibodies has led to the term "antiseptic paint," used to describe the mucus barrier to the gastrointestinal tract (13). In addition to its affinity for secretory component, the unique polymeric structure of primary secretory antibodies renders them much more efficient in agglutinating intestinal antigens. It has been estimated that agglutinating capacity of dimeric A is several times greater than comparable amounts of monomeric IgA obtained from the secretion (14).

Several recent investigations have provided direct evidence for the immune exclusion function of intestinal antibodies. Williams and Gibbons (15) examined the adherence properties of oral pathogens (Streptococcus viridans) to epithelial cell surfaces before and after exposure of these organisms to specific secretory IgA antibodies. They observed a definite decrease in adhesion of these bacteria to the cell surface after exposure to secretory antibodies. They concluded that secretory IgA antibodies block specific binding sites on the bacterial cell wall and thereby interfere with bacterial adherence to epithelial surfaces. A decrease in adherence results in decreased colonization as well as enhanced clearance of the bacteria by oral secretions. Additional studies have shown interference in the attachment of Vibrio cholerae to intestinal mucosa by secretory IgA intestinal antibodies (16). The presence or absence of intestinal antibodies capable of interfering with specific bacterial adherence may also be important in determining the nature of indigenous gut bacterial flora.

Intestinal antibodies can also protect against the effects of toxic bacterial by-products (e.g., enterotoxins). Secretory antitoxins complexing with cholera toxin can prevent the toxin's binding to receptors on intestinal microvillus membranes and thereby interfere with the activation of adenylate cyclase, a necessary step in the active secretion associated with toxigenic diarrhea. In like manner intestinal antibodies interfere with the uptake of nonviable antigens introduced directly into the gastrointestinal tract (17). We have previously reported that intestinal antigens become rapidly associated with antibodies present in the glycocalyx. Antigen–antibody complex formation at that site appears to prevent migration of antigen to the cellular membrane surface and thereby to interfere with pinocytosis by enterocytes. Other investigators have demonstrated that IgA myeloma antibodies injected into the respiratory tract of laboratory animals interfere with the uptake of human serum albumin by respiratory epithelium (18).

In addition to the direct effect of mucosal antibodies on intestinal antigens, the formation of immune complexes on the intestinal surface may facilitate other important nonimmunologic protective mechanisms that can further contribute to immune exclusion of antigen from the mucosal surface. We have reported that a formation of antigen–antibody complexes on the gut surface results in enhanced degradation of antigens retained within the glycocalyx (19). Using pancreatic duct ligation experiments, we showed that the enhanced breakdown of antigen–antibody complexes was mediated by pancreatic enzymes adsorbed to the mucus coat lining the surface of the gut. Complexing of antigens by antibodies present in the mucus layer allowed for prolonged retention of antigens in that compartment coating the cell surface. At that site degradation of antigen by pancreatic enzymes adherent to the mucus coat could proceed. More recently, antigen–antibody complexes, formed in antibody excess, have been shown to stimulate the release of mucus from goblet cells of the mucosa. Release of mucus may in turn "wash" the intestinal surface free of complexes and thereby further interfere with the access of antigen to the epithelial cell (20).

## DERANGEMENT IN GASTROINTESTINAL STRUCTURE AND FUNCTION IN PRIMARY MALNUTRITION

Having briefly reviewed the normal intestinal adaptations to the external environment primarily with respect to the development and maintenance of the crypt–villus unit as a basis for providing a mucosal barrier of defense, this section will explore some of the derangements in gastrointestinal structure and function that have been reported in association with both experimental and clinical malnutrition. The changes are listed in Table 1. The basic defect that develops is a relative decrease in mature

**Table 1    Gastrointestinal Changes in Malnutrition**

---

Subtotal villous atrophy
Decreased functional surface area
Disrupted mucosal barrier
  ↓ enzymes
  ↓ antibodies
  ↓ mucins

Decreased crypt cell turnover
  ↓ migration of cells
  ↓ mitosis
Altered intestinal flora
Relative pancreatic insufficiency

---

surface area because of decreased cell proliferation, migration, and maturation within the crypt–villus unit. This derangement in gastrointestinal structure results in a significant decrease in absorption of nutrients as part of the end stages of digestion and transport as well as lessening the effectiveness of the mucosal barrier protection provided by the microvillus and glycocalyx. As a result of decreased energy available for normal cell turnover, migration, and maturation, the intestine can no longer operate optimally as either a digestive organ or an organ of protection. The consequence of this development may contribute to the secondary manifestations of the disease (infection, allergic reactions, etc.) associated with primary malnutrition.

In general, the information depicted in this section is a composite of reports from the literature describing malnutrition. Because of variability in degrees of malnutrition, that is, marasmus versus kwashiorkor, the spectrum of gastrointestinal dysfunction reported is considerable. Patients who have severe protein-calorie malnutrition (kwashiorkor) are those who have the most abnormal intestinal morphologic changes and the most functional disruption. In contrast to this, individuals who have primarily calorie deficiency (marasmus) without concomitant protein malnutrition may have what appears to be a normal intestine with minimal dysfunction. Furthermore, data reported from experimental animal studies are difficult to interpret because the basis for producing malnutrition varies from animal to animal and from experimental design to experimental design. These results, therefore, provide a very confusing spectrum of malnutritional states from which a wide variety of gastrointestinal changes have been described. In general, however, morphologic and functional changes occur even after short periods of decreased nutri-

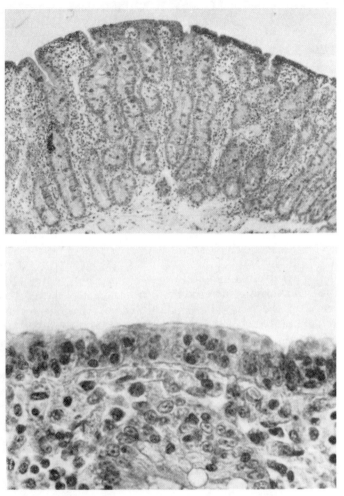

**Figure 3.** Flattened mucosa similar to celiac disease in kwashiorkor. *Top,* low power to show absence of villi and flat surface. There is moderate infiltration of the lamina propria with lymphocytes and plasma cells. P.A.S. stain. *Bottom,* high power to show low surface epithelium with irregularly distributed nuclei. The brush border is irregular and sparse. H. and E. stain. [From O. Brunser, A. Reid, F. Monckeberg, et al., Jejunal biopsies in infant malnutrition: With special reference to mitotic index, *Pediatrics,* 38, 608, (1966).]

tional intake. These changes may either persist and worsen or rapidly reverse, depending on the state of the patient's nutritional rehabilitation. This observation is particularly true in patients who are rehabilitated by using enteric sources of nutrients, a subject that will be discussed in more detail later.

## Morphologic Changes in Malnutrition

Several comprehensive review articles have been written to describe the morphologic changes in association with malnourished conditions (21– 23). In general, the changes in morphology of the small intestine differ strikingly in patients manifesting marasmus compared to those with kwashiorkor. Figure 3 depicts the appearance of the small intestine in a patient with classic kwashiorkor disease. This representative biopsy specimen shows subtotal atrophy of the villus and a shortening of crypts; at higher magnification one notes striking changes in the epithelial cells lining the villus. Instead of the columnar epithelial cell with a well-developed microvillus membrane and glycocalyx which is the usual end result of maturation of cells migrating up the crypt into the villus, one sees a cuboidal cell type which has a disrupted microvillus and very little evidence of glycocalyx, suggesting a severe disruption in the differentiation and maturational process of cells geared for both protection and function within the gastrointestinal tract. In contrast to the histologic appearance of the small intestine of patients with protein-calorie malnutrition (kwashiorkor), patients with marasmus have very little evidence of abnormality at the light microscopic level and have some minor abnormalities of epithelial cells at the ultrastructural magnification. Again, in this condition the microvilli are decreased in number and glycocalyx fails to develop completely. In general, the morphologic changes in both conditions respond very quickly to nutritional rehabilitation; obviously the more severely malnourished patients respond more slowly than the less severely affected. If one uses the "mitotic index," that is, the percentage of epithelial cells from the crypt of Lieberkuhns in mitosis expressed numerically as a percent of total epithelial cells in the entire crypt–villus unit, one sees a striking decrease in cell turnover in both kwashiorkor and marasmus, suggesting that cellular proliferation is strikingly decreased under these conditions of malnutrition (24). Brown and co-workers (25) have looked at the incorporation of [3]H-thymidine with autoradiographic techniques and have demonstrated that even after a short period of decreased nutritional intake in experimental animals, there is a considerable difference in the number of labeled cells present within the crypt as well as in the migration of labeled cells from the crypt into the villus. This observation suggests that with both short-term and long-term malnutrition, the cell turnover and migration rate is disrupted as a result of a decrease in availability of nutrients (25). In additional studies reported in experimental animals it has also been demonstrated that if one compares the amount of brush border enzyme as measured by sucrase in small intestinal homogenates to the amount of crypt enzyme as measured by thymidine kinase in small intestinal homogenates, a striking decrease in the available mature surface area is noted (21).

## Functional Abnormalities

In addition to morphologic changes that are apparent in patients with malnutrition, several important gastrointestinal functions are disrupted. These include the production of hydrochloric acid within the stomach, causing a decrease in the gastric acidity and loss of gastric barrier to bacteria (26). In addition, pancreatic insufficiency has been demonstrated under conditions of severe malnutrition (27). Furthermore, alterations in the end stages of digestion at the membrane level and a concomitant decrease in absorption of nutrients have been noted (28). Barbezate and Hansen (29) have observed that both resting and stimulated pancreatic enzyme levels, including lipase, trypsin, chymotrypsin, and amylase, are generally decreased in malnourished states. These studies would strongly suggest that under conditions of severe malnutrition pancreatic function is severely impaired. This impairment would alter intraluminal digestion and further contribute to the maldigestion–malabsorption problems accompanying malnutrition. Several lines of evidence suggest that absorption at the epithelial level is also disrupted in malnutrition. These data, including studies by Bowie and co-workers (30), showed decrease in lactose absorption and decreased lactase levels in mucosal biopsies of children with protein-calorie malnutrition. James and co-workers (28) have reported defective sucrase hydrolysis in the intestine of malnourished individuals, and others have shown that D-xylose absorption has been decreased significantly during the clinical stages of severe malnutrition (31).

In addition to these functional changes, it is apparent that the proliferation of pathologic bacteria within the intestine is enhanced in severe malnutrition (32). With the absence of a gastric barrier, bacteria can easily gain entrance to the small intestine, colonize at the site, and produce symptoms of bacterial overgrowth syndromes. In the absence of appropriate intraluminal digestion and absorption, and with the result-

**Table 2   Immunologic Changes in Malnutrition**

---

Humoral

    Decreased SIgA

    Increased serum IgA

    Normal IgG, IgM

Cellular

    Normal absolute lymphocytes

    Decreased functional lymphocytes

      Decreased delayed hypersensitivity

      Decreased mitogen stimulation

---

ing excessive cellular debris, substrate is available for further bacterial proliferation. It is also suggested that with severe structural derangement in the intestinal tract, the proliferation of excessive numbers of bacteria may result in secondary infection within the intestine and concomitant gram negative septicemia, both frequent secondary complications of protein-calorie malnutrition.

In summary, numerous gastrointestinal alterations in both morphology and function have been described as a result of primary malnutrition. Generally, the morphologic disruption is directly related to the degree of malnutrition. Reversal of morphologic changes as a result of nutritional rehabilitation is slower than recovery from functional derangements. The functional derangement is manifested by alterations in gastric barrier, decrease in pancreatic enzyme production and release, as well as an alteration in membrane digestion and absorption. These changes contribute to the vicious cycle created in malnourished patients, which results in further malnutrition, resulting in yet further gastrointestinal dysfunction, leading to total inanition.

## IMMUNOLOGIC ABNORMALITIES IN PRIMARY MALNUTRITION

An enormous literature has accumulated describing immunologic and host defense abnormalities in association with malnutrition. A composite of this literaure is listed in Table 2. The immunologic changes shown in this table have been consistently reported both in human subjects studied clinically and in experimental malnutritional studies. As with gastrointestinal dysfunction associated with primary malnutrition, it is difficult to summarize immunologic changes because the methods of creating experimental animal models differ among investigators and the relative degree of malnutrition is associated with relative degrees of immunologic incompetence. Again, there are several excellent reviews summarizing this subject in detail (33–35).

## Humoral Abnormalities

In general, the systemic immune response manifested as levels of serum gamma globulin in patients with severe protein-calorie malnutrition are either normal or increased. The systemic antibody response in the malnourished state when increased has been attributed to excessive penetration of antigens from the mucosal surface of disrupted intestine into the circulation (36). It is felt that lymphocytes committed to immunoglobulin production, that is, B lymphocytes, are disrupted only under conditions of severe malnutrition, and generally malnutrition has very little effect on the subpopulation of lymphocyte function. In contrast to total immunoglobulin levels, serum IgA is consistently elevated in all forms of malnutrition and is directly associated with the degree of gastrointestinal morphologic and functional disruption occurring in the individual patient (36). Levels of IgG are usually normal or slightly elevated, whereas IgM and other antibody levels seem to be within the normal range. It is the consensus of the literature that the humoral immune system is in general not disrupted in malnutrition and in fact may be stimulated to produce excessive quantities of circulating antibodies, which prevent foreign antigens from gaining access to the systemic circulation across mucosal surfaces.

## Secretory Immune Response

In contrast to the systemic immune response, the secretory immune response may be severely impaired in patients with moderate to severe malnutrition. In several reported studies, the levels of secretory immune globulin A in saliva and intestinal secretions are consistently decreased in patients with protein-calorie malnutrition (37, 38). These levels return to normal after the patients have been nutritionally rehabilitated. Although the basis for discrepancy between decreased secretory IgA levels and increased serum IgA level is not known, it is postulated that the disruption of the cellular epithelium of the gastrointestinal tract in malnutrition and an associated decrease in available secretory component, the glycoprotein necessary for the transport of secretory immune globulin A from the plasma cells in the lamina propria up into the intestinal sur-

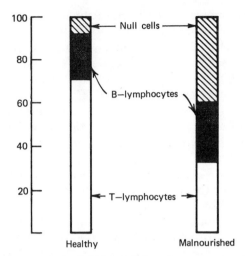

**Figure 4.** The relative proportion of T and B lymphocytes and null cells in healthy and malnourished children. [From Chandra (38).]

face, may account for this observation. In general, as the epithelium surface improves with rehabilitation so do the levels of secretory immunoglobulin A. Based on our earlier discussion of SIgA function in secretions, it would seem likely that a deficit of SIgA is an important contributing factor to the severe derangement in host defenses within the gastrointestinal tract. In fact, SIgA deficiency probably accounts for the enhanced penetration of mucosal barrier by bacteria, toxins, and intestinal antigens. Further implications of this derangement in humoral responsiveness will be discussed later.

## Cellular Abnormalities

An enormous literature has accumulated describing various abnormalities of cell-mediated immune (CMI) responsiveness in primary malnutrition. In general, the number of circulating lymphocytes in patients with malnutrition has not been reported to be abnormal. Chandra has claimed that the distribution of lymphocytes is altered in malnourished individuals (38). He reports an increased number of null lymphocytes, nonfunctional lymphocytes, compared to T lymphocytes and B lymphocytes (38). This observation would suggest that there is a maturational delay in lymphocytes or a decrease in the response of precurser lymphocytes to be committed to either T or B lymphocyte function. Figure 4 depicts the comparative degree of abnormality in lymphocytes in patients with malnutrition versus normal controls.

Whereas the number of circulating lymphocytes in patients with malnutrition appears to be normal, the ability of these lymphocytes to respond to stimulation is severely impaired. As one assesses CMI from a functional standpoint, it is apparent that delayed hypersensitivity, as manifested by skin testing and PHA stimulation, is decreased in patients with protein-calorie malnutrition (39). The ability for lymphocytes to form E rosettes is also impaired in this condition (39). The implication from these studies is that CMI activity at the functional level is impaired in patients with protein-calorie malnutrition. Just as with humoral immunologic abnormalities, the cellular immune responsiveness quickly returns to normal during periods of nutritional rehabilitation. Patients who are maintained in the hospital under adequate caloric intake will quickly revert to normal responsiveness, as manifested by delayed hypersensitivity in skin testing, PHA stimulation, and E rosette formation (40). To what degree disruption in cell-mediated immunity contributes to the decreased postresponsiveness of patients with malnutrition is not known. It would appear that the increased susceptibility to infections, particularly those that are controlled by T lymphocytes, has been noted.

### Phagocytosis in Malnutrition

Just as abnormalities have been noted in other components of host defense, the capacity for polymorphonuclear neutrophils to phagocytose bacteria is disrupted in protein-calorie malnutrition. In several studies, it has been demonstrated that organisms may be engulfed by phagocytes but the time during which these cells are killed is severely impaired. This would suggest a decrease in the capacity of circulating phagocytes to adequately police the systemic circulation against potential systemic infection. This abnormality, coupled with those previously described, can account for the marked increases in susceptibility to infection noted in patients with protein-calorie malnutrition (41).

### CONSEQUENCES OF HOST DEFENSE ABNORMALITIES IN MALNUTRITION

Having briefly reviewed the current concepts, basic mechanisms of host defense within the gastrointestinal tract, and the abnormalities incurred in gastrointestinal morphology, function, and host defense in primary malnutrition, I would like to consider briefly the consequences of disruption in local host defense in the gastrointestinal tract in primary malnutrition. Figure 5 depicts the pathologic state of macromolecular

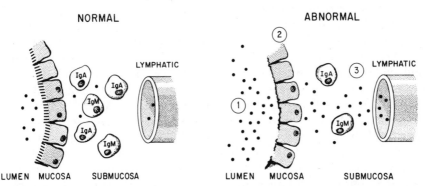

**Figure 5.** Physiologic and pathologic transport of antigens across the intestinal mucosal barrier into the systemic circulation. *Left,* Under normal conditions, factors within the intestinal lumen, on the surface of the epithelial cells, and within the lamina propria combine to limit the access of antigens to the systemic circulation. *Right,* However, when these natural defenses are disrupted, excessive quantities of antigenic material may enter the circulation and contribute to clinical diseases. Factors contributing to pathologic absorption of antigens include (1) decreased intraluminal digestion, (2) disrupted mucosal barrier, or (3) decrease in IgA-producing plasma cells in the lamina propria. [From Walker (8).]

transport when structural and functional abnormalities in the intestine interfere with local host defenses. As a result of an altered intestinal barrier that occurs in primary malnutrition, excessive quantities of intestinal antigens, toxins, and microorganisms can gain access to the intestinal interstitium and enter the portal circulation. Host defenses within the interstitium and in the systemic circulation are insufficient to control this penetration of macromolecules. As a result, clinical secondary complications develop, such as bacterial gastroenteritis, septicemia, and immune complex–immunologically mediated disease processes involving vital organs such as the liver and kidneys. Although these statements are in part speculation, several observations have been noted in malnourished patients which would suggest that secondary disease processes can occur and contribute to the overall morbidity of malnutritional states (2).

Both direct and indirect evidence has been reported to suggest that as a consequence of protein-calorie malnutrition there is a disruption of the mucosal barrier and pathologic uptake of intestinal antigens. Chandra (42) reported an increase in circulating food antibodies in patients admitted to his hospital with severe malnutrition. He noted that a highly significant number of these patients had circulating hemoagglutination antibodies against milk proteins and other food antigens. This indirect evidence suggests that these protein antigens are not being appropriately digested within the gastrointestinal tract and are free to cross a disrupted mucosal surface and enter the systemic circulation, perhaps to evoke a systemic immune response. Although there may not be a direct correlation between the levels of hemoagglutination antibodies to food proteins and evidence of allergic or immunologic disease in these individuals, this observation reflects the general disruption of a mucosal barrier and suggests that potentially dangerous antigens can gain access to the host. Experimentally, Worthington (43) has shown that in severely protein malnourished animals there is direct histochemical evidence of increased uptake of protein enzymes into intestinal epithelial cells. In our laboratory, we have preliminary evidence to suggest that radiolabeled antigens can be transmitted in larger quantities from the intestine into the circulation of animals subjected to severe protein-calorie malnutrition than in controls. These studies provide direct evidence that the mucosal barrier has been altered as a result of malnutrition and that intestinal macromolecules can be absorbed in pathologic quantities under these conditions.

Although no studies have been done that directly investigate bacterial adherence to the intestinal surface of malnourished animals, one can draw indirect conclusions from the comparison of the intestinal tract of the immature infant with that of the malnourished individual. In both conditions, there is a relative decrease in mature surface area and increase in immature nondifferentiated epithelial cells. It has been demonstrated in the immature intestine containing an increase in undifferentiated surface area that intestinal bacteria, particularly E. coli, can adhere more avidly to the intestinal surface (44). As mentioned earlier, adherence of bacteria to the intestinal surface determines the bacteria's ability to proliferate within the intestine, and is a factor in controlling the nature of the flora within the gastrointestinal tract. It would seem reasonable, therefore, to assume that similar processes are occurring in the gastrointestinal tract of malnourished individuals. If this were true, this might account for the increased susceptibility to both local intestinal bacterial gastroenteritis and systemic gram-negative septicemia. These studies at this point are speculative, but may be confirmed as new experimental models develop to investigate the association between malnutrition and bacterial proliferation.

In like fashion, it has been demonstrated that enterotoxins adhere avidly to receptor sites on the surface of the intestinal tract and that the immature intestine seems to be more susceptible to the effects of the toxin than the more mature intestinal tract (45). Under these circumstances it would seem reasonable to assume that enterotoxins released from bacterial flora within the intestinal tract may have a more devastating effect on the malnourished patient than on the normal individual. It is difficult to separate the defect in the clinical setting, since most individuals subject to toxigenic diarrhea are already malnourished. Again, this area must be investigated from a research standpoint and information from these studies can be very helpful in our attempts to control consequences of host defense abnormalities within the gastrointestinal tract.

In summary, we have suggested that as a result of a disrupted mucosal barrier, an important function of the gastrointestinal tract, individuals with protein-calorie malnutrition develop an increased uptake of intestinal antigens which can contribute to secondary disease processes as part of the spectrum of dysfunctions associated with this condition. These individuals, in turn, are more vulnerable to uptake of microorganisms from the intestinal tract, the toxic by-products of these microorganisms, and potentially dangerous and sensitizing proteins ingested or elaborated from bacteria within the intestine.

As a result of pathologic uptake of macromolecules, secondary conditions such as bacterial gastroenteritis, gram-negative septicemia, and systemic immunologic responses may create secondary disease states which contribute to the overall poor prognosis of malnutrition. If attempts are made to counteract these secondary manifestations by providing passive protection or active intervention against intestinal antigens, the severity of protein-calorie malnutrition may be lessened. Considerably more research and clinical trials must be done before information will become available to answer these questions.


## THE IMPORTANCE OF NUTRITIONAL REHABILITATION IN GUT HOST DEFENSE

The goal in the treatment of patients with primary malnutrition is to rehabilitate these patients as quickly and safely as possible to the point where their own bodies' natural defenses are appropriate in dealing with potential dangers of infection and allergic reaction. This is accomplished by a coordinated effort involving the use of extensive information from other forms of clinical and experimental research studies. In general, the use of nutrients enterically is preferred to bypassing the intestine by such means as total parenteral nutrition. The consequences of enteric supplementation are particularly important to the rapid repair of the mucosal barrier.

In general, it is appropriate to consider a combination of parenteral alimentation, providing calories that are directly given to the systemic circulation, and enteral alimentation, gradually utilizing the gut in its primary role as a digestive and absorptive organ. An extensive literature has accumulated over the last several years to suggest that if the intestinal tract is bypassed as part of the rehabilitation process, there will be a much slower recovery of morphology and function noted in the malnutrition and in host defense abnormalities that have been previously discussed. In general, the use of enteric feeding provides direct access of nutrients to epithelial cells, allowing for more rapid differentiation in turnover and reversal of the abnormalities noted. It also stimulates enteric hormones, which have been demonstrated in experimental settings to be trophic in nature, and facilitate the rapid maturation of the intestinal tract.

Human colostrum may potentially and theoretically be used to provide passive protection during the critical period of additional rehabilitation. It has been demonstrated in young infants with immature and vulnerable small intestines that this viable substance provides cells and antibodies as well as antibacterial substances which can help coat the intestinal surface and provide a passive immune barrier until the active barrier can develop adequately. This might be something to consider in the future in our treatment of severely malnourished patients, particularly those who are young infants and might utilize colostrum more effectively.

In summary, an important adaptation of the gastrointestinal tract to the extrauterine environment is its development of a mucosal barrier against the penetration of harmful substances (bacteria, toxins, and antigens) present within the intestinal lumen. In its functional state, the gut must be prepared to deal with and control bacterial colonization, dispose of toxic byproducts of bacteria and viruses (enterotoxins and endotoxins), and withstand the continuous ingestion of antigens (milk proteins). These potentially noxious substances, if allowed to penetrate the mucosal epithelial barrier under pathologic conditions, can cause inflammatory and allergic reactions which may result in gastrointestinal and systemic disease states.

To combat the potential danger of invasion across the mucosal barrier, the gut has developed an elaborate system of defense mechanisms within the lumen and on the luminal mucosal surface which act to control and maintain the epithelium as an impermeable barrier to uptake of macromolecular antigens. These defenses include a unique local immunologic system adapted to function in the complicated milieu of the intestine as well as other nonimmunologic processes, such as the gastric barrier, intestinal surface secretions, peristaltic movement, and natural antibacterial substances (lysozyme, bile salts), which also help to provide maximum protection for the intestinal surface.

Unfortunately, during malnutritional states, particularly in severe protein-calorie malnutrition, this elaborate local defense system is disrupted. As a result of the disruption of the mucosal barrier, malnourished patients are particularly vulnerable to pathologic penetration by harmful intraluminal substances. The consequences of altered defense are susceptibility to infection and potential for hypersensitivity reactions and for formation of immune complexes. With these reactions comes the potential for developing life-threatening diseases, such as bacterial gastroenteritis, sepsis, and vital organ failure (liver and kidney). If measures are rapidly taken to rehabilitate the malnourished individual, disruptions in gastrointestinal defenses are quickly repaired and no secondary diseases develop to complicate the patient's clinical condition. For optimum response within the gastrointestinal tract, enteric feedings must be instituted rather than utilizing total parenteral nutrition as the only source of calories.

In this review of intestinal defenses in malnutrition, the factors that contribute to the development of a protective mucosal barrier have been discussed and the specific defects in gastrointestinal and immunologic function in malnutrition have been presented. The short- and long-term implications of a defective mucosal barrier in malnutrition with respect to disease states have also been considered.

# REFERENCES

1. W. A. Walker and K. J. Isselbacher, *Gastroenterology*, **67**, 531 (1974).
2. W. A. Walker, *Pediatrics*, **57**, 901 (1976).
3. L. D. Dworkin, G. M. Levine, N. J. Farber, and M. H. Spector, *Gastroenterology*, **71**, 626 (1976).
4. L. R. Johnson, E. M. Copeland, S. J. Dudrick, L. M. Lichtenberger, and G. A. Castro, *Gastroenterology*, **68**, 1177 (1975).
5. P. Sunshine, J. J. Herbst, O. Kedorsky, et al., *Ann. N.Y. Acad. Sci.*, **176**, 16 (1971).
6. J. J. Herbst and P. Sunshine, *Pediat. Res.*, **3**, 27 (1969).
7. I. Antonowicz and E. Lebenthal, *Gastroenterology*, **72**, 1299 (1977).
8. W. A. Walker, *Ped. Clin. N. Am.*, **22**, 731 (1975).
9. R. M. Rothberg, *J. Pediat.*, **75**, 391 (1969).
10. E. J. Eastham, T. Lichauco, M. I. Grady, and W. A. Walker, *J. Pediatr.*, **93**, 561 (1978).
11. B. Kletter, I. Gray, and S. Freier, *Int. Arch. Allergy Appl. Immunol.*, **40**, 656 (1971).
12. W. A. Walker and K. J. Isselbacher, *New Engl. J. Med.*, **297**, 767 (1977).
13. J. Bienenstock, *Prog. Immunol.*, **4**, 197 (1974).
14. M. E. Lamm, *Adv. Immunol.*, **22**, 223 (1976).

15. R. C. Williams and R. J. Gibbon, *Science,* **177,** 697 (1972).

16. E. S. Fubura and R. Freter, *J. Immunol.,* **111,** 395 (1973).

17. W. A. Walker, K. J. Isselbacher, and K. J. Bloch, *Science,* **177,** 608 (1972).

18. T. B. Tomasi, Jr., *The Immune System of Secretions,* Prentice-Hall, Englewood Cliffs, N.J., 1976.

19. W. A. Walker, S. N. Abel, M. Wu, and K. J. Bloch, *J. Immunol.,* **117,** 1028 (1976).

20. W. A. Walker, M. Wu, and K. J. Bloch, *Science,* **175,** 370 (1977).

21. F. E. Viteri and R. E. Schneider, *Med. Clin. N. Am.,* **58,** 1487 (1974).

22. O. Brunser, *Clin. Gastro.,* **6,** 341 (1977).

23. R. M. Suskind, *Ped. Clin. N. Am.,* **22,** 873 (1975).

24. E. Duque, O. Bolanos, H. Lotero, and L. G. Mayoral, *Am. J. Clin. Nut.,* **28,** 901 (1975).

25. H. O. Brown, M. L. Levine, and M. Kipkin, *Am. J. Physiol.,* **205,** 868 (1963).

26. M. Gracey, D. E. Stone, M. D. Suharjono, et al., *Am. J. Clin. Nutr.,* **27,** 345 (1974).

27. M. D. Thompson and H. C. Frowell, *Lancet,* **1,** 1031 (1952).

28. W. P. T. James, *Lancet,* **1,** 333 (1968).

29. G. O. Barbezat and J. D. L. Hansen, *Pediatrics,* **42,** 77 (1968).

30. M. D. Bowie, G. L. Brickman, and J. D. L. Hansen, *J. Pediat.,* **66,** 1083 (1965).

31. C. T. Gurson and G. Saner, *Helvet. Ped. Acta.,* **24,** 510 (1969).

32. L. J. Mata, F. Jimenez, M. Cordon, et al., *Am. J. Clin. Nutr.,* **25,** 1118 (1972).

33. R. M. Suskind, in *Malnutrition and the Immune Response,* R. M. Suskind, Ed., Raven Press, New York, 1977, p. 169.

34. C. G. Neumann, G. J. Lawlor, E. R. Stiehn, et al., *Am. J. Clin. Nut.,* **28,** 89 (1975).

35. R. Suskind, S. Sirishmha, V. Vithayasai, et al., *Am. J. Clin. Nut.,* **29,** 836 (1976).

36. R. K. Chandra, in *Malnutrition and the Immune Response,* R. M. Suskind, Ed., Raven Press, New York, 1977, p. 155.

37. S. Sirishinha, R. Suskind, R. Edelman, et al., *Pediatrics,* **55,** 166 (1975).

38. R. K. Chandra in *Malnutrition and the Immune Response,* R. M. Suskind, Ed., Raven Press, New York, 1977, p. 113.

39. C. G. Neumann, E. R. Stiehn, M. Swenseid, et al., in *Malnutrition and the Immune Response,* R. M. Suskind, Ed., Raven Press, New York, 1977, p. 81.

40. P. Kulapongs, R. M. Suskind, V. Vithayasai, et al., in *Malnutrition and the Immune Response,* R. M. Suskind, Ed., Raven Press, New York, 1977, p. 101.

41. S. D. Douglas and K. Schopfer, in *Malnutrition and the Immune Response,* R. M. Suskind, Ed., Raven Press, New York, 1977, p. 235.

42. R. K. Chandra, *Arch Dis. Child.,* **50,** 532 (1975).

43. B. S. Worthington, E. S. Boatman, and C. E. Kenny, *Am. J. Clin. Nutr.,* **25,** 1118 (1972).

44. M. Hirshberger, D. Mirelman, and M. M. Thaler, *Ped. Res.,* **11,** 500 (1977).

45. E. S. Fubura and R. Freter, *J. Immunol.,* **111,** 395 (1973).

# Index

**219**